Coconut Therapy for Pets

By
Bruce Fife, ND

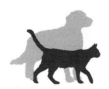

Piccadilly Books, Ltd.
Colorado Springs, CO

Every effort has been made to ensure that the information contained in this book is complete and accurate. However, neither the publisher nor the author is engaged in rendering professional advice or services to the individual reader. The ideas, procedures, and suggestions contained in this book are not intended as a substitute for consulting with your veterinarian. All matters regarding your pet's health require veterinary supervision. Neither the publisher nor the author are responsible for your pet's specific health or allergy needs that may require veterinary supervision and are not responsible for any adverse reactions to the recipes or procedures contained in this book.

Acknowledgements
We would like to thank Charisa Antigua of CocoTherapy and all the many other people who contributed photographs, testimonies, and stories for this book. Grateful acknowledgement is given to Wikipedia for the photos on pages 25, 70, 72, 77,78, and 158.

Piccadilly Books, Ltd.
P.O. Box 25203
Colorado Springs, CO 80936, USA
info@piccadillybooks.com
www.piccadillybooks.com

Library of Congress Cataloging-in-Publication Data

Fife, Bruce, 1952-
  Coconut therapy for pets / by Bruce Fife, ND.
    pages cm
  Includes bibliographical references and index.
  ISBN 978-0-941599-95-5 (paperback)
  1. Pets--Health. 2. Pets--Diseases--Alternative treatment. 3. Coconut oil--Therapeutic use. 4. Coconut oil--Health aspects. I. Title.
  SF745.5.F54 2013
  636.088'7--dc23
                                    2013033307
Published in the USA

Contents

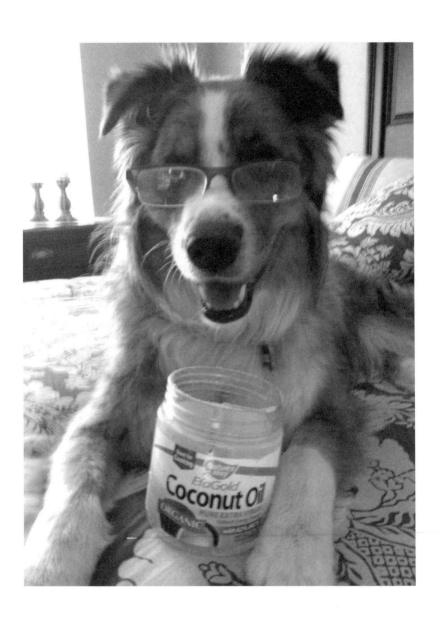

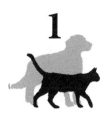

1

The Miracle of Coconut Oil

COCONUT OIL TO THE RESCUE

If you go into any major pet store you will see a large number of products designed to treat various common health issues. You will find shampoos, sprays, supplements, and medications of all types for the purpose of treating bad breath and body odor, fleas and ticks, intestinal worms, dry or itchy skin, dull coats, skin rashes, ear mites, injuries and wounds, eye problems, digestive complaints, liver issues, and joint problems; the list can go on and on. Often the products don't work very well or else you need to continue with the treatment for an extended period of time to keep the condition at bay. You could easily spend $100 to $200 a month or more on these types of products. But you don't have to. Most of these conditions can easily and successfully be treated with just one inexpensive product—coconut oil. For a fraction of the cost, coconut oil can solve most of these issues and do a far better job of it. But you need not take my word for it. Read for yourself what pet owners are saying about coconut oil.

"My cat had tapeworms," says Mary Jo. "When I started giving her coconut oil they vanished almost immediately."

"I have used virgin coconut oil on my dog's eyes when they get 'icky,'" says Cireena, "and it really clears it out."

"My dog *loves* coconut oil!" says Ruth. "She has allergy and skin problems and in the past had a bad doggy smell. She now gets coconut oil twice a day and her skin problems and odor have disappeared! She loves it! She licks her bowl clean as well as the spoon that I use to put the oil into her bowl."

"My horse had some kind of irritation on its face," says Lori. "I've been putting virgin coconut oil on it almost every day and it is definitely clearing."

Coconut oil has proven to be so beneficial to animals that owners are giving it to their pets as a dietary supplement. Some manufacturers are now adding it into their dietary supplements and pet foods. One of these is PowerStance for horses. "The last 5 months I have noticed an immense change in my horses' appearance, performance, and overall attitude," says Callie. "Everyone that sees my horses wants to know what they are on because they look so great! The only supplement I feed them is PowerStance! Coconut oil is the key. I love my horses' glowing coat and I know they love feeling so good."

"We hear about a host of canine health problems here at Life on the Leash," says Victoria Schade, APDT certified pet dog trainer and author of *Bonding with Your Dog*. "Flaky skin, hot spots, yeasty ears, dull smelly coats, infected cuts, cracked paws…it's not pretty. Once we determine that the maladies aren't related to diet (sub-par dog foods can contribute to the issues listed above), I suggest the next best line of defense: coconut oil."

A SUPERFOOD

Many people are surprised to learn that coconut oil can offer so many health benefits to their pets. Coconut is a nutritious food that possesses both nutritional and medicinal properties. It is a superfood—a food that provides substantial health benefits beyond its nutrient and calorie content. Although coconut and coconut oil have been viewed primarily as food for humans, animals love it and can benefit from it too.

I first discovered the remarkable health benefits of coconut years ago after a colleague said to me, "Coconut oil is one of the *good* fats." I was shocked. Coconut oil is high in saturated fat, and at the time I believed that all saturated fats were bad because I was told they promoted heart disease. My colleague cited some studies to back up her statement, and I was intrigued. I wanted to learn more. I wanted to know how coconut oil could be healthy even though it was highly saturated. To find my answer, I went to the medical literature to see what researchers were actually learning about coconut oil. I wanted the cold hard facts from medical research, not unfounded myths based on prejudice and fragmented information or marketing hype you often see spouted in magazine articles and diet books.

As I read through the medical studies I was amazed at all of the health benefits associated with coconut, especially coconut oil. I learned that coconut oil is uniquely different from other dietary fats. It is composed primarily of a special group of fat molecules (fatty acids) called medium chain fatty acids (MCFAs). Most of the fats in our diet consist of long chain fatty acids (LCFAs). This makes coconut oil unique and gives the oil its remarkable nutritional and medicinal properties.

All fats and oils are composed of triglycerides, of which there are many different types. Coconut oil is composed predominately of medium chain triglycerides (MCTs). When we eat coconut oil, our bodies break down the MCTs into individual MCFAs. You will see the terms MCTs and MCFAs used in research papers, food and supplement labels, the Internet, etc. If this explanation sounds too confusing to you, that's ok. All you need to know is that MCFAs come from MCTs which come from coconut oil. People often use the terms MCFAs and MCTs interchangeably.

In my research, I learned that MCFAs from coconut oil were used extensively in hospitals to treat critically ill patients. The fatty acids were included in IV solutions and feeding tube formulas because studies show that patients recover faster when they receive them. Coconut oil is much easier to digest than other fats, so it has been used by doctors to treat a number of malabsorption syndromes in children and adults. Newborn infants are routinely given formula containing MCFAs or coconut oil. Studies have shown that infants, particularly premature infants, have a higher survival rate and grow faster if given MCFAs. In fact, coconut oil or MCFAs have been added to all brands of commercial infant formula for decades to capitalize on the health-promoting properties these fats provide.

What are some of the health benefits of MCFAs? For one, they possess potent antimicrobial properties capable of fighting off disease-causing bacteria, viruses, fungi, yeast, and parasites, without causing any harm to infants or to us. They can help moderate sugar release and thus help balance blood sugar levels, which can ease symptoms associated with diabetes. They possess anti-cancer properties. They provide a quick and easy source of energy which can boost metabolism and aid in weight management. They have antioxidant effects, are anti-inflammatory, and boost immune function. They can improve over-all health and well-being. And, contrary to popular misconceptions about saturated fat, coconut oil causes no harm to the heart or arteries, but acts as a heart tonic and improves heart function.

I began using coconut oil myself and recommending it to others. I've seen it clear up hemorrhoids, stop bladder infections, remove cancerous skin lesions, help people lose excess weight, boost their energy levels, and overcome a multitude of diverse health conditions. I was so impressed with all the health benefits associated with coconut oil that I felt compelled to write a book detailing these facts, which I titled *The Coconut Oil Miracle*. In this book, I describe many of the health properties identified in published medical research as well as historical data and my own personal experiences.

SAFE FOR PETS

After the publication of *The Coconut Oil Miracle,* I started to receive emails and letters from people asking me if it was safe to give coconut oil to dogs, cats and other pets. My answer: "Of course!" Virtually every health benefit associated with coconut oil in humans is applicable to animals. In fact, much of what we know about the health aspects of coconut oil was first observed in animals.

Whether you agree with it or not, animals are often used in medical and nutritional research. Fortunately for the animals, coconut oil has demonstrated to be protective and beneficial in these studies. It is from this research that we learned of coconut oil's anticancer properties. When researchers fed coconut oil to lab animals or applied it onto their skin, the animals didn't get cancer. We know that coconut oil neutralizes a variety of toxins because animals are protected from these poisons if given the oil. Studies found that coconut oil can help heal the digestive disorders, like

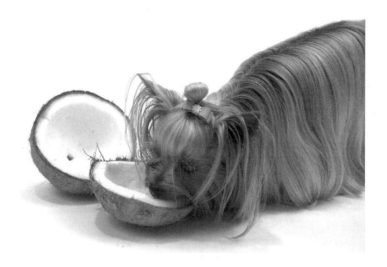

ulcerative colitis, because it does so in animals.[1] Animal studies also demonstrate how and why coconut oil digests easier than other oils and how it is converted into energy rather than body fat. The antiviral, antibacterial, and antifungal effects of coconut oil have been demonstrated in animals. Whether the researchers used rats, mice, dogs, sheep, chickens, cows, or horses, coconut oil has had positive effects.

These studies have also shown that coconut oil is well tolerated, causing the animals no harm, unlike many drugs and even some dietary supplements and other treatments. In these studies, there have been no signs of harm caused by the consumption of coconut oil or MCTs. Even in toxicity studies where researchers fed enormous amounts of coconut oil to animals, there have been no adverse effects. Coconut oil is completely nontoxic even in abnormally high doses that would never occur outside a research laboratory. Coconut oil is a food, not a drug, so you don't need to worry about "overdosing." The worst thing that could happen if your dog or cat lapped up an entire jar of coconut oil is that it might experience loose stools. This would happen with the overconsumption of any type of fat or oil. You should not be too concerned about giving your pet too much coconut oil because it isn't dangerous.

Coconut oil is the richest natural source of MCFAs—the magic behind the oil. One of the few other sources of MCFAs is breast milk, of which MCFAs are an essential component. Because of the antimicrobial properties of MCFAs, infants are provided with protection against infections for the first few months of their lives while their immune systems are still developing. MCFAs are also much easier to digest than other fats, so they provide infants with a quick and easy source of nutrition. This is one of the reasons why coconut oil or MCFAs are included in all hospital and commercial infant formulas. Adding coconut oil to formula makes it more like the real thing. Human babies aren't the only ones who benefit from MCFAs. All mammals produce MCFAs in their mammary glands. These special fatty acids are important for the health, growth, and development of all mammals. This is another reason why coconut oil is not only safe for pets but can provide them many health benefits.

I have heard many comments from people over the years who have been giving their pets and farm animals coconut oil. For the most part, the animals seem to love it and readily lap it up. The most common effect reported is an improvement in their fur or hair. It becomes shinier and more youthful looking. It also freshens the breath—no more disgusting doggy breath. Energy levels improve especially in older or lethargic pets. Skin lesions and infections clear up quickly, even stubborn ones that have not responded to conventional medicines and antibiotics. Insect stings and bites, cuts, and other injuries heal quicker. Intestinal parasites are killed or expelled. Pet owners even report the success of using coconut oil for very serious conditions such as environmental poisoning, cancer, and diabetes. Coconut oil offers a simple, inexpensive, and easy remedy for many of these problems.

Keep in mind that coconut oil is not dangerous so you don't need a doctor or veterinarian to give you permission to use it. Unless you see a holistic veterinarian, he or she will probably know little about coconut oil and out of fear of saturated fat may tell you not to use it. But it can do no harm. It is good for your pet and can be used internally and externally.

Coconut oil has been used successfully to treat a wide variety of health problems in humans. It can be just as successful with animals. Some of the benefits of coconut oil for pets and other animals are listed here.

Given Orally:

- Improves the health and appearance of the skin and coat in mammals
- Improves the health and appearance of the skin and feathers in birds
- Reduces or eliminates body odor and bad breath
- Improves energy and balances metabolism
- Promotes healthy thyroid function
- Helps reduce excess body fat and maintain proper weight
- Prevents and fights bacterial, viral, and yeast infections
- Improves immune function
- Helps relive kennel cough
- Improves oral health and whitens teeth (can use as a toothpaste)
- Helps ease allergy symptoms
- Eases inflammation
- Sooths itchy or irritated skin
- Improves digestion and nutrient absorption
- Protects against digestive disorders such as ulcers and colitis
- Expels or kills parasites
- Helps balance blood sugar and alleviate symptoms associated with diabetes
- Reduces risk of cancer
- Promotes good nerve and brain function and prevents dementia
- Helps build strong bones
- Helps prevent and ease arthritis and ligament problems
- Improves overall health and well-being

Applied Topically:

- Speeds healing from cuts, burns, insect bites and stings, and other injuries
- Disinfects wounds
- Helps clear up skin conditions such as rashes, eczema, contact dermatitis, flaky skin, skin infections, hot spots, and abnormal growths
- Helps clear up ear and eye infections
- Protects against fleas, ticks, mites, and other parasites
- Acts as a coat conditioner and deodorizer
- Sooths and heals dry, cracked paws and elbow calluses

Although I will mention a few notable studies in the following chapters, I'm not going to bore you with a lot of scientific details or go into long explanations as to how and why coconut oil can stop or reverse all these conditions. If you are interested, you can learn the science behind it in my other books such as *The Coconut Oil Miracle* and *Coconut Cures*. You can also find more of the science on my website at www.coconutresearchcenter.org. The book you are reading now is meant to be a guidebook rather than a scientific text. In the following pages, I let pet owners tell their own stories and share their experiences using coconut oil and other coconut products. These personal accounts are sometimes more revealing than formal studies, more practical, and usually more interesting, yet all of these cases are backed by sound, scientific evidence.

You may hear some skeptics claim that coconut oil has not been tested adequately enough to demonstrate that it is effective in treating health problems in animals or that its safety is unknown and could make the condition worse. Most conventional veterinarians who are not familiar with natural cures are likely to say this. They do so as an excuse to discourage the use of coconut oil. Unfortunately, their more expensive, "scientifically proven" chemical drugs often don't work as well as expected and generally have toxic side effects. There is a lot of research backing the use of coconut oil. Unlike drugs, coconut oil has no toxic side effects and is completely safe. The real test of its effectiveness is to try it yourself and see how it works. Many people have already done so and have been fully satisfied with the results.

2

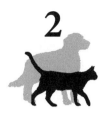

The Importance of Dietary Fat

THE LOW-FAT MYTH

True or false: the less fat there is in the diet the healthier it is? Most people would probably say this statement is true. The correct answer, however, is false. Too little fat in the diet can lead to severe nutritional deficiencies. Fat, believe it or not, is an essential nutrient. We, as well as our pets, must have an adequate amount of fat in our diets for proper growth and development and to obtain and maintain good health.

Over the past couple of decades fat has been unjustly criticized as the primary cause of our rising obesity rates as well as a contributing factor in heart disease, diabetes, cancer and just about every other illness imaginable. Everywhere we turn, we are cautioned about limiting our fat intake. After years of being fed low-fat propaganda, we are led to believe that if a low-fat diet is good, a very-low fat diet must be better, and a no-fat diet must be best of all. The low-fat myth extends through all corners of our society. Even our children think this way. In a poll conducted among schoolchildren, an incredible 81 percent thought that the healthiest diet possible was one that eliminated all dietary fat. Such a diet, however, would be a nutritional disaster.

We have been following low-fat guidelines now for nearly three decades, but we are fatter and sicker than ever. Even though total fat consumption has declined, overweight and obesity rates have skyrocketed. Degenerative disease is at an all-time high. Heart disease is still our number one killer. Diabetes, cancer, Alzheimer's and other diseases continue to rise. Reducing the fat in our diet has not helped; in fact, it may have made matters worse. Diet studies have consistently shown that low-carb, moderate- to high-fat diets are superior to low-fat or low-calorie diets for weight loss. Studies also show that the higher the fat content of the diet, the greater the weight loss. The problem with expanding waistlines is not due to eating too much fat, but to eating too much carbohydrate—sugar, sweets, and grain products. Nonetheless, many people find it hard to change ingrained beliefs and continue to beat the drum of cutting fat consumption. Your own doctor or veterinarian may be among this group.

This anti-fat hysteria has spilled over into the formulations and recommendations of pet foods. As a consequence, our pets' diets are generally fat deficient. This is one of the reasons why pets nowadays are experiencing increasingly higher rates of degenerative disease and ill health. Veterinarians like to claim that the increase in conditions associated with old age is because our pets are living longer now. Our pets certainly outlive their wild cousins, that's for sure, but that is because they don't have to compete for food and battle the elements every day of their lives just to survive. However, domesticated dogs and cats don't live any longer now than they did 50 or 60 years ago. In fact, dogs' and cats' lifespans have actually decreased despite great advances in veterinary medicine.

Anyone who is suffering from osteoporosis, arthritis, gout, fibromyalgia, diabetes, irritable bowel syndrome, infertility, multiple sclerosis, chronic fatigue syndrome, stroke, Alzheimer's, Parkinson's, ALS, depression, and in fact, most any neurological problem is most likely either fat deficient or eating the wrong types of fats. The same is true for people who experience multiple infections or illnesses every year and those who suffer from nutritional deficiencies. Nutritional deficiencies, particularly subclinical or marginal deficiencies, are especially troubling because they aren't always easy to recognize and the symptoms are often misinterpreted as signs of normal aging. Likewise, many of the health problems our pets face may be caused, at least in part, by a lack of good quality dietary fats.

WHY FAT IS IMPORTANT
Building Blocks

Fat comprises the primary structural component of every cell in your body. Fats make up the cell membrane—the skin that holds the cells together. The cells in your heart, lungs, kidneys, muscles, and every other organ are dependent on fat to hold them together. Your brain is composed of 60 percent fat and cholesterol.

Dietary fats, including cholesterol, are used not only to make structural components of cells, but also to make the hormones and prostaglandins that control and regulate bodily functions and play important roles in maintaining chemical balances within the body. Vitamin D, estrogen, progesterone, testosterone, DHEA, and many other hormones are constructed out of cholesterol. Even cholesterol is made from fat. Hormones are the main regulators of metabolism, growth and development, reproduction, and many other processes. Likewise, prostaglandins, which are hormone-like substances made from fat, influence blood lipid concentrations, blood clot formation, blood pressure, immune response, and inflammation response to injury and infection.

A diet lacking in fat can seriously reduce the efficiency of your immune system and thus make you more susceptible to disease. The immune system not only protects us from infectious illnesses but from many degenerative conditions as well. Life would be impossible without fat.

Cells, prostaglandins, and hormones are constantly being created and destroyed. Since fat is used for so many purposes throughout the body, it makes sense that we need to consume an adequate amount of fat daily in order to supply the building blocks for new tissues and hormones. This is especially true for those who are rapidly growing and those who are very physically active. This is why adequate fat is critically essential for the proper growth and development of children and young animals.

Energy Source

Gasoline powers cars; fat powers our bodies. Fat is one of the three energy-producing nutrients. The other two are protein and carbohydrate. Our bodies use fat as a source of energy to power metabolic processes and maintain life. At least 60 percent of the body's energy needs are supplied by fat.

Every cell in our bodies must have a continual source of energy to function properly and maintain life. The body's first choice of fuel is glucose, which can be derived from either carbohydrate or protein. When there is adequate carbohydrate or protein in the diet to meet energy needs, fat is put into storage inside fat cells. Excess carbohydrate and protein are converted into fat and also packed away into fat cells for use later. Between meals or during times of low food intake, fat is pulled out of storage and used to supply the body's ongoing energy needs.

Fat provides more calories per gram than either carbohydrate or protein because it is a compact energy source that can be stored away and used later. Energy is measured in terms of calories. The body can store more calories (i.e., energy) per gram with fat than it can with either carbohydrate or protein. If the body stored protein instead of fat, you would look like a bloated pork sausage because your storage cells would have to double in size to accommodate energy demands. So be thankful your body stores fat and not protein.

Between meals and during prolonged periods of fasting, if you don't have fat or adequate amounts of fat stored in fat cells, your body will resort to using protein, such as muscle tissue, for energy. Your body will literally consume itself to get the energy it needs to stay alive.

Essential Fatty Acids

Fats are composed of individual fat molecules called fatty acids. There are many types of fatty acids. Two families of fatty acids, known as omega-3 and omega-6 fatty acids, are considered absolutely necessary for good health. They are referred to as *essential fatty acids* or EFAs. They are classified as essential because the body cannot make them from other nutrients. We must get them from our foods. These essential fatty acids are found in varying amounts in all foods—meat, fish, vegetables, nuts, seeds, as well as vegetable oils and animal fats. Avoiding or removing fats from foods decreases these essential nutrients and can lead to EFA deficiency.

EFAs are important in the diet for making the hormone-like substances, prostaglandins. Prostaglandins influence blood fat concentrations, blood clot formation, blood pressure, immune response and inflammation response to injury and infection, and play important roles in maintaining chemical balances within the body. Without these fats the body suffers from deficiency disease symptoms that include skin lesions, neurological and visual problems, growth retardation, reproductive failure, skin abnormalities, and kidney and liver disorders.

EFAs are found in most vegetable oils but are often damaged by refining and processing or destroyed by free radicals. Exposure to heat, oxygen, and light quickly destroy (oxidize) the EFAs, making them useless. Therefore, conventionally processed vegetable oils, which are exposed to all these conditions, are inferior sources for EFAs. Likewise, the EFAs in highly processed foods (including dry and canned pet foods) will also be oxidized and pretty much useless.

Medium chain fatty acids (MCFAs), like those found in coconut oil, are considered to be *conditionally essential*, that is, under certain circumstances they are just as important to get in the diet as other essential fatty acids. MCFAs are essential during pregnancy and early growth and development. For this reason, MCFAs are found in the milk of all mammals, including humans. MCFAs are also needed for various malabsorption syndromes where EFAs and other fats are not well tolerated or absorbed.

While coconut oil supplies only a small percentage of EFAs, one benefit to using coconut oil in the daily diet is that the MCFAs work synergistically with the essential fatty acids, improving the way the body uses these fats. A diet rich in coconut oil can enhance the efficiency of essential fatty acids by as much as 100 percent! Not only that, but coconut oil also acts as antioxidant, protecting EFAs from destructive oxidation inside the body. If the diet includes an adequate amount of coconut oil, the need for EFAs is substantially reduced. Therefore, if the diet is low in EFAs, adding coconut oil can help prevent EFA deficiency.

Nutritional Source

It's a mistake to think of fat as a poison. On the contrary, fat is a necessary nutrient just as much as protein, vitamin C, or calcium. Without fat in our diet, we would all sicken and die from nutrient deficiencies.

Low-fat foods are actually detrimental because they prevent complete digestion of food and limit nutrient absorption. Fat is necessary for the proper digestion and absorption of many essential nutrients. Fats slow down the movement of food through the stomach and digestive system. This allows more time for foods to bathe in stomach acids and be in contact with digestive enzymes. As a consequence, more nutrients, especially minerals which are normally tightly bound to other compounds, are released from the foods and absorbed into the body.

Low-fat foods can promote mineral deficiencies. Calcium, for example, needs fat for proper absorption. For this reason, low-fat diets encourage osteoporosis and joint problems. It is interesting that people often avoid eating fat as much as possible, choosing non-fat or low-fat milk, yet by consuming reduced-fat milks, the person fails to effectively absorb the calcium. This may be one of the reasons why people can drink loads of milk and gobble down calcium supplements to no end yet still suffer from osteoporosis.

In addition to improving the absorption of calcium and other minerals, fat also improves the absorption of amino acids (building blocks for proteins), fat soluble vitamins such as vitamins A, D, E, K, and important phytonutrients and antioxidants such as beta-carotene, CoQ10, lycopene, and others. Even the water soluble B vitamins are better absorbed when fat is present.

All fats improve vitamin, mineral, amino acid, and nutrient absorption, but coconut oil is even more effective at this than other fats. Animal studies have shown that beriberi, a potentially fatal vitamin B_1 deficiency, can be avoided even when the diet is critically deficient in vitamin B by adding coconut oil to the diet. Coconut oil does not contain vitamin B_1, but it does make what little vitamin B_1 that is present in the foods more biologically available or, in other words, more absorbable, thus preventing the deficiency disease. Coconut oil was shown to be more effective in preventing vitamin B deficiency than other fats.

Even though a food may contain ample vitamins and minerals, it is not the amount present that is important; it is the amount that is actually absorbed that is important. Pet foods may claim to meet certain minimum levels of various nutrients, but if they are not completely absorbed, they do little good. Studies show that adding fat to vegetables increases the absorption of vitamins by up to 18 times! Just adding fat to foods can seriously improve the nutrient content. Using adequate fat is one of the keys to achieving a complete and balanced diet.

Other Benefits

Fat has many important functions in the body. I have not mentioned all of them, just enough to show you how important they are in the diet. Researchers are discovering more benefits of dietary fat all the time. For example, in a study done at the University of Buffalo in 1999, female soccer players were able to perform longer at a higher intensity on diets composed of 35 percent fat rather than on diets of 27 percent or 24 percent fat. This study showed that higher-fat diets boost athletic performance. In another study, military pilots were shown to have quicker reaction times, clearer thinking, and better overall performance under stress if they were fed a high-fat diet.[1]

Fat also helps regulate digestion and absorption of blood sugar, thus helping to prevent insulin resistance and diabetes. Without adequate amounts of fat in the diet, blood sugar levels can go out of control after eating a carbohydrate-rich meal.

Fat helps satisfy hunger longer so you don't feel the need to eat as often, thus helping you to eat fewer calories. Eating fat helps you *lose* weight.

As you can see, fat is a very important component of our food. It is just as important for our pets. It is involved in a variety of functions throughout the body, many of which science has yet to fully understand.

BAD FATS

Hydrogenated Fats

Dietary fats are not all alike. There are many different types of fats and each has a different effect on the body. Modern processing and food manufacturing have created some fats that are detrimental to health and contribute to weight gain and other health problems. In general, the more processing a fat or oil has undergone and the older it is, the less healthy it is.

19

Fake fats like margarine, shortening, and other hydrogenated vegetable oils are the most processed and the least healthy. When vegetable oils are hydrogenated, natural fatty acids are transformed into what are called trans fatty acids. The trans fatty acids that are created this way are unnatural; they are fake fats that cause havoc in the body. The body doesn't recognize them as food but does identify them as some type of fat and so tries to use them like it does with any other type of fat. However trans fatty acids don't function like natural fats and cause a great deal of trouble. Trans fats have been linked to heart disease and circulatory problems, diabetes, and autoimmune disorders.

Hydrogenated vegetable oils are common food additives and are found in many processed foods. You should never feed your pets any human or animal food that contains hydrogenated vegetable oils. Read the ingredient label and look for the words "hydrogenated" or "partially-hydrogenated" vegetable oil.

Oxidized Fats

Any oil that has undergone extensive processing is potentially harmful. Exposure to heat, oxygen, and light has an adverse effect on oils, causing them to oxidize or, in other words, become rancid. Rancidity is a form of decay. When iron oxidizes or decays, it turns into rust. When oils oxidize they become rancid. If you put a carton of pasteurized milk on the countertop at room temperature and let it sit there for several days, it will begin to rot and become putrid. While the milk sits on the countertop, the heat (even room temperature), oxygen, and what little light the milk is exposed to attack the milk fats. These fats oxidize, becoming rancid. They, in turn, cause proteins to oxidize. It's the rotting proteins in the milk that creates the awful smell.

The fatty acids that make up the fats and oils in the diet can be grouped into three major categories: saturated, monounsaturated, and polyunsaturated. All vegetable oils and animal fats consist of a mixture of these three groups of fatty acids. To say an oil is saturated or monounsaturated is grossly oversimplifying. No oil is purely saturated or polyunsaturated. Olive oil, for example, is often called "monounsaturated" because it is *predominantly* monounsaturated, but, like all vegetable oils, it also contains some polyunsaturated and saturated fat. Beef fat, as well, contains saturated, monounsaturated, and polyunsaturated fatty acids.

Oils that have a high percentage of saturated fats, like coconut oil, are naturally very stable and highly resistant to oxidation. Oils high in polyunsaturated fats, like corn and soybean oils, are highly unstable and are very vulnerable to oxidation; consequently, they have a short shelf life. Polyunsaturated vegetable oils oxidize ten times faster than saturated fats when exposed to the same conditions (heat, oxygen, light). In fact, oxidation of polyunsaturated vegetable oils starts in the factory at the very moment the seeds or grains are first crushed to extract the oils. As time goes on, oxidation continues. When oils are added to unrefrigerated foods, such as dry pet food, these oils are exposed to heat, oxygen, and light for several months, causing them to become highly rancid. Even relatively stable animal fats become rancid.

The primary problem with rancidity is that the oxidation of oils causes the formation of free radicals. Free radicals are damaged, highly unstable, reactive molecules that attack nearby molecules, causing them to become free radicals as well. This causes a chain reaction, resulting in the creation of thousands of destructive free radicals.

In the body, free radicals attack our cells, literally ripping their protective membranes apart. Sensitive cellular components like the nucleus and DNA, which carry the genetic blueprint of the cell, can be damaged, leading to cellular mutations or death. A living cell attacked by free radicals degenerates and becomes dysfunctional.

The more free radicals that attack our cells, the greater the damage and the greater the potential for serious destruction. If the cells that are damaged are in our heart or arteries, what happens? If they are in the brain, what happens? If they are in our joints, pancreas, intestines, liver, or kidneys, what happens? Think about it. If the cells become damaged, dysfunctional, or die, can these organs fulfill their intended purpose?

Free-radical damage has been linked to the loss of tissue integrity and to physical degeneration. As cells are bombarded by free radicals, the tissues become progressively impaired. There are many sources of free radicals in our environment and it is impossible to avoid them completely. Some researchers believe that free-radical destruction is the actual cause of aging. The older the body gets, the more damage it sustains from a lifetime accumulation of attack from free radicals.

When unsaturated oils oxidize (go rancid), they generate free radicals. The more unsaturated an oil is, the more easily it oxidizes. Therefore, polyunsaturated oils are much more vulnerable to oxidation than monounsaturated oils, and monounsaturated oils are much more vulnerable than saturated oils.

Oxidized Cholesterol

Technically, cholesterol is not a fat because it is not composed of fatty acids, but since it is similar in character, it is often referred to as a fat. Contrary to popular belief, cholesterol is not the evil substance it is often made out to be. It is an essential component of our bodies. Cholesterol is an important structural component in all of our cells; it is used to make vitamin D, bile, and many of our hormones. It is a major component of nerve and brain tissue. Cholesterol is far more important to our health than most people realize.

Years ago cholesterol feeding studies in animals suggested that eating too much cholesterol could promote the development of atherosclerosis (plaque buildup in the arteries). It was believed that atherosclerosis could build up to the point that it would block the flow of blood to the heart and cause a heart attack. This idea lead to the cholesterol hypothesis of heart disease, that high blood cholesterol levels increase the risk of heart disease.

It was in the 1970s that researchers discovered that dietary cholesterol existed in two distinct forms: oxidized and reduced. In fresh, natural foods, cholesterol occurs in the harmless reduced form. This is the type of cholesterol that makes up the majority of our brain tissue and is used as a component of cell membranes; it is not found in human arterial plaque. The type of cholesterol that builds up in the arteries is oxidized cholesterol along with oxidized fatty acids. These are the only types of fats found in plaque.[2]

Cholesterol, like fatty acids, can become oxidized. Oxidation damages cholesterol, making it harmful. Only the oxidized form is toxic to arteries.[3-4] Natural, unadulterated cholesterol is not harmful to the arteries and cannot initiate or promote heart disease.[5] Cholesterol must be oxidized before it can cause atherosclerosis in artery walls.[6]

A large number of published studies support the fact that oxidized fats (both cholesterol and fatty acids) are far more harmful to arterial health than natural fats. Therefore, cholesterol is now viewed as harmless unless it becomes oxidized.[7]

When it was discovered that only oxidized fat is involved in the generation of arterial plaque, researchers became curious enough to repeat the original rabbit-feeding studies that established the cholesterol hypothesis. They suspected that the first researchers put the fat-rich food into cages and left it for the rabbits to eat throughout the day. This allowed the fat on the surface of the food to react with the oxygen in the air and become oxidized. Oxygen, sunlight, and heat (even room temperature) can initiate rancidity and free-radical reactions.

When researchers repeating these experiments made efforts to protect the fat in the food from oxidizing, the animals' arteries remained healthy. The fat content of the food was increased and the rabbits' blood cholesterol went as high as 1,500 to 2,000 mg/dl—ten times the upper limit currently considered acceptable for humans—but no fatty deposits formed! So even in vegetarian animals, natural cholesterol is harmless.

Today, researchers intentionally add oxidized cholesterol to animal diets in order to study atherosclerosis. This, unfortunately, has lead to a lot of confusion regarding fat and cholesterol. On the Internet, coconut oil critics will often claim that this oil is harmful because it causes heart disease. To prove their point they will cite rabbit and hamster feeding studies where oxidized cholesterol was added to coconut oil and fed to the animals. Invariably the animals developed atherosclerosis. The mistake they make is to claim that it was the coconut oil in the animals' diet that caused the atherosclerosis. Coconut oil and other fats are routinely used in such studies with oxidized cholesterol. The oxidized cholesterol is in a powdered form and must be dissolved in some type of fat to be fed to the test animals. When oxidized cholesterol is added to fat—any type of fat—it causes atherosclerosis. It doesn't' matter if they use coconut oil, soybean oil, canola oil, olive oil or any other type of oil, the combination of oxidized cholesterol and oil will cause atherosclerosis. It is not the coconut oil causing the problem, because any oil will do the same. It is the oxidized cholesterol that is the culprit. When these studies are repeated, without the use of oxidized cholesterol, coconut oil and other fats do not cause atherosclerosis.

Oxidized cholesterol or fatty acids, because they involve the formation of destructive free radicals, can damage arterial walls. Studies with rabbits show that those fed oxidized cholesterol have damage, while those fed normal cholesterol don't.[8] What we know now is that it's not the total level of fat or cholesterol in the blood that's important, but the amount of oxidized fat and oxidized cholesterol that is the issue. Many people with relatively low blood fat levels develop cardiovascular disease because a large amount of this fat is oxidized. Others who have high-cholesterol readings do not experience cardiovascular disease because the fat in their blood is normal, that is, not oxidized.

Coconut oil is very stable and highly resistant to oxidation even when exposed to heat, oxygen, and light. For this reason, it makes a good cooking oil. You can be assured that coconut oil is perfectly safe to feed to your pets whether they are carnivores or vegetarians. The same cannot be said about the fats and cholesterol in many of the commercial pet foods on the market however. Unfortunately, most pet foods, particularly dried foods, contain both oxidized oils and oxidized cholesterol.

FAT DEFICIENCY

Dietary fats are just as important to your pet's health as they are to yours. Commercial pet foods are sorely deficient in good fats. Much of the fat they do contain is rancid and therefore of little value. As a consequence, many pets are fat deficient. "This is the most common nutritional deficiency I see in my practice," says Karen Becker, DVM. "The symptoms I encounter on a daily basis include cats with dry skin and chronic oral inflammation, and dogs with recurrent skin and ear infections." Cats and dogs are not the only pets affected by fat deficiencies; ferrets, rabbits, hamsters, horses, and birds of all types would do a lot better if they had more fat in their diets.

Adding a high quality source of fat can bring about improved health. Coconut oil is an excellent source of fat that can not only satisfy most fat requirements but can provide many additional health benefits beyond what you would get from other fats.

Coconut oil can have remarkable effects on your pet's overall health and quality of life. Foods given to herbivorous animals are especially fat deficient. Horses, for example, tend to get very little fat in their diets even though fat is a required nutrient, particularly for working horses that need the additional calories. Dr. Dan Moore, a practicing holistic veterinarian, says, "...horses, in general, don't get enough fat, and get far too much sugar from sweet feed and corn...the best source in my opinion, is coconut oil...coconut oil is stable, and much less likely to go rancid than flax or rice bran source.

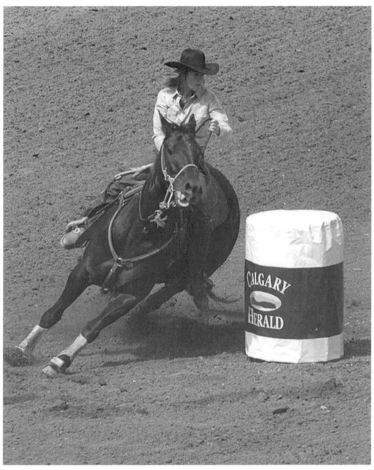

Barrel racing is a rodeo event in which a horse and rider attempt to complete a clover-leaf pattern around a set of barrels in the fastest time.

Vegetable oil and corn oil are practically useless except for calories, which most horses get way too much of anyway."[9]

In Australia, coconut meal and coconut oil are commonly added to the feed of competitive horses. Horse owners there have discovered that the addition of coconut products improves their horses' racing times, performance, and appearance. Horse owners in the United States and Canada have taken notice and are now adding coconut products into their own horses' feed.

A scrawny, sorry-looking young horse in upstate New York was rejected by its original owner because of its poor health. He was named "Dollar" because that was all he was worth. The horse had a condition known as "cribbing." Cribbing is an abnormal, compulsive behavior characterized by biting stall doors or fence rails, arching the neck, and sucking in air. It is linked to higher incidences of stomach ulcers and colic and is believed to be caused by nutritional deficiencies.

"My daughter got into barrel racing two years ago and bought her first horse 'Dollar' for $10," says Stacey Sontag. "The previous owner did not want him because he was a cribber and we were told he would never be faster than a 20 second horse…he looked very sad when we got him. His coat and eyes had no shine, he did not have any energy, and was never excited." Following the advice of a friend, they began to supplement his feed with coconut oil. "Within a couple weeks his eyes were brighter and within a month his coat was glistening…My daughter is now running low 16's on him and he doesn't seem to get as tired anymore."[10] Within a year, Dollar went from a reject to a money-winning race horse with the aid of coconut oil. It is amazing what the addition of fat, particularly coconut oil, can have on the health of many animals.

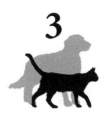

3

Animals Love Coconut

THE TASTE OF COCONUT OIL

Pretty much all forms of wildlife love the taste of coconut. In coconut growing areas of the world, wild hogs, dogs, birds, reptiles, and insects feast on coconut whenever they can get it. One creature that has taken the eating of coconuts to an extraordinary level is a crustacean known as the coconut crab. The coconut crab has such powerful claws that can rip through the fibrous husk, crack open the hard shell, and feast on the tasty meat inside. Although coconut crabs eat a variety of foods, they relish coconuts so much that they will actually climb dozens of feet up the trunk of the coconut palm to harvest the delicious fruit at the top. They must really like it if they go to that much trouble to get it.

Domestic animals love it too. Dogs, cats, guinea pigs, gerbils, mice, rabbits, birds, and even farm animals such as chickens, horses, cows, pigs, and goats will readily eat coconut if given the opportunity. They recognize it as a nourishing food.

It is not only a nutritious food but a superfood with special health-promoting properties. Many pet owners use it like they would a dietary supplement to enhance and enrich the nutritional quality of their pet's diet. Often the nutrients in food are not effectively absorbed into the body but go in and come out of the digestive tract providing absolutely no benefit. Coconut oil enhances nutrient absorption. In addition to the improved nutrition, coconut oil also

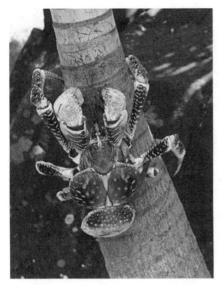

provides health-promoting medium chain fatty acids. Most of the incredible health properties associated with coconut come from these unique fatty acids.

It wouldn't matter how healthy coconut oil is if your pet won't eat it. If the taste was disagreeable, even hiding it in your pet's food may not work. Fortunately, most animals love the taste of coconut. Unlike vitamins and medications that pets will often refuse to eat, pet owners find their animals relish the taste of coconut and coconut

Coconut crab climbing the trunk of a coconut palm to harvest the fruit.

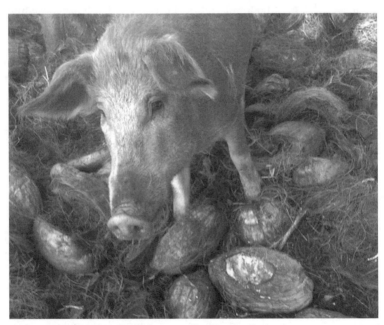

A pig enjoying his daily ration of coconut fruit.

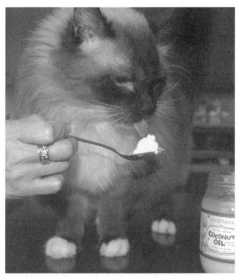

Most pets love the taste of coconut.

oil and readily eat it. In fact, you can hide less tasteful vitamins and medications in the coconut oil and your pet will lap it up without complaint. Dogs and cats love the taste of coconut and many will lick it off a spoon. It can be fed as is or mixed in their food. A typical reaction is, "I tried adding coconut oil to my cat's food this evening and she loved it—licked the bowl clean!" Many others share similar experiences with coconut oil or virgin coconut oil (VCO).

I have started my Italian greyhound on the oil for about one month. Her coat is improving every day and she no longer has flaky skin. She absolutely LOVES her daily coco treat.
Erica Kremer

My late Rusty absolutely LOVED Cocotherapy. After he got so sick with the brain tumor especially, it seemed to liven him up and give him more energy. Molly loves Cocotherapy because it's great for her allergies and itchy skin. Plus I can hide her other supplements in it and she laps it right up. I have noticed a decrease in her itching and scratching and an increase in her energy level since giving her coconut.
Heather Collins

My dog Max, a Brittany spaniel, will actually stop eating his food when he sees me reaching for the coconut oil. He sits and waits for me to dish it out. I've never before seen a dog stop eating voluntarily and wait for something like that.
Chrissy L.

My dog Sophy loves the coconut oil so much, she snatched it off the counter and ate about a cup of it before I could catch her and get it back.

Frances

I just drop a dollop in their food, or sometimes I let them lick off the spoon. All three of my dogs would chew your face off for it. They love it.

R. D.

I seriously busted out laughing about how coconut oil is like crack cocaine for dogs. That's so true. My puppy will come running when she hears the jar open. I run the jar under warm water. A little bit will begin to melt. I pour what's melted over her morning meal. I probably give her about a tablespoon a day.

K. L.

Oh, my little Maltese dog loves the VCO (virgin coconut oil). Whenever I put it on he will run up and lick my leg, or if I am holding him he will lick my hands. Sometimes I put a little in the dog's food, and his food is gone in seconds!

A. B.

We give our cat about a teaspoon a day of virgin coconut oil. She loves it. In fact, when we open the jar just to use some for ourselves, she'll come running!

T. W.

I started giving my two female cats coconut oil a few years back when after using it on my face they would lick my fingers. So I checked it out online and all was a go so I gave them a little at a time. They loved it but will only eat as much or little as they want. It's helped with hairballs and pooping, and gives a beautiful shiny coat.

Lisa K.

Dogs and cats aren't the only animals that go crazy over coconut. Horses, birds, and other animals love it too. Cocosoya, mentioned below, is a commercially prepared dietary supplement sold to horse owners that is a combination of coconut and soybean oils.

I feed Cocosoya oil and I LOVE, LOVE, LOVE IT!! It is so much bang for your buck. Plus the horses love it too. They will eat ANYTHING as long as it has Cocosoya oil on top of it and I have some picky eaters in the barn. Their coats are shiny and hooves are in great shape.

J. J. R.

The horses really do like the coconut oil! We are having to feed our horses hay cubes to prepare them for a week at a horse ranch where all they feed is hay cubes. My daughter's horse particularly, does not like the cubes! I suggested to her to put some coconut oil on them to see if they would help him eat the cubes and it worked! He started eating them. My only concern now is being able to afford the coconut oil for both our horses and us!

Mary

With our birds, it's organic coconut oil!...With coconut oil, some of our birds eat wee bits from a spoon (in its solid form). Our GW (greenwing macaw) would eat it all day every day if I let him. He loves it! So does our Amazon (parrot).

Doris

FRESH AND DRIED COCONUT

It is not just the oil that pets like but the coconut meat as well. Pets will devour fresh or dried coconut if given the opportunity. You can give them the coconut meat from a fresh coconut or give them dried coconut. Avoid the sweetened desiccated coconut you get at the grocery store. It is loaded with sugar as well as preservatives. At your local health food store or online, you can purchase unsweetened coconut flakes or desiccated coconut. This is the same product you would buy to use in baking for your own use. If it's good enough for humans, it should be good enough for your pet. One company called CocoTherapy produces a product called Coconut Chips especially for pets. These are unsweetened slices of dried coconut. The chips are high in fiber, free of sugar, salt, and other additives and make a great alternative to over processed pet treats containing artificial ingredients and preservatives. Dogs love them.

Both fresh coconut and dried coconut contain a high percentage of coconut oil. Fresh coconut is about 33 percent fat (in the form of coconut oil). Pets can get many of the same health benefits they get from coconut oil by eating the meat.

I bought the oil and chips for my dogs...even though my dogs didn't really have any health problems. My dogs go batties for it! I didn't think my cat would like any of it, because she's very picky, but to my surprise, she LOVES the chips! She even sniffs the oil in my hands and takes little licks. At first she was hesitant, then it started to grow on her... now she actually comes running when she hears me open the jar. She used to have little sores/blisters around her mouth, and was on and off prednisone, which I hate. Since she's been eating the chips and oil the sores are drying up and disappearing. I've stopped the prednisone, and I'm so happy she seems to be getting better. Originally, I got the oil and chips for my dogs, little did I know that my cat would love it too, and it would help the sores in her mouth.
Shelley Williams

We have three cats...the two youngest ones go crazy for the chips! When we open up the container we store the chips in, they come RUNNING from wherever they are in the house! The older one loves the oil...we've noticed a big change in his coat since he started taking it.
Jim Jones

There have been times when my dogs have gotten diarrhea, and I have found that shredded coconut seems to help bind the stools, and my dogs love it. I just hand feed it to them, and they gobble it up.
Connie

Coconut meat in the shell can make a novel treat and chew toy. One dog owner says, "I was pleasantly surprised to notice the recreational value of a cut-in-half coconut for my dogs. It meant hours of happy gnawing until the last bit of meat was out of it and lots of fun thereafter as a toy." A piece of coconut shell with the meat still attached is like a bone with residual meat still hanging on. It cleans

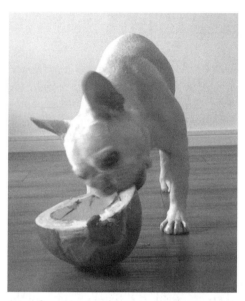
Murphy enjoying his coconut in the shell.

dogs' teeth and gives them the benefits of coconut meat and oil.

Some people give full unopened coconuts to their dogs to play with. The round coconut provides dogs exercise as they chase it around and pounce upon it like they were in the wild taking down prey. Coconuts can take a real beating and if they break open they can be gnawed on and the meat eaten without problem. This can provide the dogs with hours of entertainment and exercise. This is definitely an outside activity though. The round coconuts can scoot around in any direction and may cause damage hitting into the living room wall or end table. Plus, the water inside would make a mess once the shell is cracked. You might want to crack the coconut slightly with a hammer to drain the liquid and to make it a little easier for your dog to open the rest of the way.

Dogs love to chew. Chewing lets a dog know what things feel and taste like, and whether it's good to eat. It's a natural part of being a dog and an important part of a dog's early development. Just like babies, pups chew to soothe sore gums when teething. It can take up to a year for a pup's adult teeth to come in. Some dogs remain very active chewers all their lives. If a dog does not have something to chew, he may take it upon himself to find something, like a good shoe or a new baseball glove. Destructive chewing is common in dogs who spend a lot of time alone, since it's a way of fending off boredom or anxiety. A coconut shell with the meat provides an excellent way for dogs to satisfy their inborn urge to chew without resorting to your clothes and personal items.

Dogs aren't the only animals that like to chew coconuts. Apparently even horses like to join in on the fun.

I find coconut milk or even coconut water is fantastic for coats, has a ton of vitamins and minerals, and is much cheaper than the oil. When we were racing in Florida, we would get whole coconuts (green with the husks still on) and put the whole thing in the stall. The horses loved chewing on them and the fiber off the husks is great, and they would eat the whole coconut and they LOVED the water inside. We did this at least once a week or so and the horses looked great.
N. R.

COCONUT MILK AND WATER

The terms coconut milk and coconut water are at times used interchangeably. However, there is a distinct difference between the two. Coconut water is the liquid that is naturally found inside the cavity of a fresh coconut. When you pick up one of the brown hairy coconuts at the grocery store and shake it, the sound you hear is the swishing of the coconut water. Coconut milk, on the other hand, is extracted from coconut by shredding and squeezing the liquid out of the meat. The juice that comes out of the meat is coconut milk. Coconut water and coconut milk look and taste completely different. Coconut water is a relatively clear liquid that looks much like ordinary water. Coconut milk is a thick, creamy white liquid that resembles dairy milk or cream.

Coconut water is a good source of vitamins, minerals, amino acids, and antioxidants. It is essentially fat-free, meaning it contains no coconut oil, yet it still provides many health benefits. Research has shown that in humans it can help reduce high blood pressure, protect against cancer, aid digestive function, relieve constipation, reduce risk of heart disease, improve blood circulation, prevent atherosclerosis, and enhance immune function. Because it is a good source of essential electrolytes, it has become popular as an oral rehydration beverage. When we perspire, we lose electrolytes (mineral ions) such as sodium and potassium. Drinking coconut water can replenish these electrolytes and keep us hydrated. For this reason, coconut water is known as "Nature's Gatorade." However, coconut water is superior to Gatorade as a rehydration beverage. It provides better rehydration with no chemical additives. You can learn more about the many health benefits of coconut water from my book *Coconut Water for Health and Healing*.

Coconut water has a slightly sweet, subtle flavor. Strangely, it doesn't taste much like coconut. It has a flavor all its own. You can purchase coconut water in a variety of containers—cans, cartons, glass. The most common is 11 ounce Tetra Pak cartons. Of course, you can also get coconut water from a fresh coconut, which is the best source, and the most tasteful.

Coconut water can help rehydrate our pets as well as us. Most pets seem to enjoy it.

My puppy, Sophie, drinks a carton of plain coconut water a day. She loves it. She gets about a 1/3 of a carton with each meal. She goes right to it after exercise. I now give coconut water to my friends with puppies. They all love it. Hard to see any direct results but I am sure it is good for her immune system, her coat, and just plain rehydration. Our vet seems to think it is a good idea. She also gets coconut oil (that will loosen her stool a little so I give her a little pumpkin or sweet potato in her food) every day. Her adult coat is coming in soft and shiny.
Barbara M.

Coconut milk has a look and consistency similar to that of dairy cream. Its nutritional profile is very different from that of coconut water. It contains a much higher percentage of protein and fiber and is loaded with coconut oil. A typical 14 ounce can contains about 5 tablespoons (70 g) of coconut oil. This is one of the reasons why coconut milk is so good; it provides another way to eat coconut oil and can provide all the health benefits of coconut oil. If your pet doesn't take to coconut oil very well, it may enjoy the milk.

Coconut milk is usually sold in 14 ounce cans. You can find it in the ethnic section of most grocery stores. Chose a brand that does not have any sugar, preservatives, or hard to pronounce chemical names in the ingredients. Do not use the coconut milk beverages sold in milk cartons found in the refrigerated dairy section of the grocery store. These products are not coconut milk, but are coconut milk *beverages* and contain little real coconut milk but a lot of water, sugar, and other additives. Your best source of coconut milk is to make it at home from fresh or dried coconut (see Chapter 12).

NOT SURE OF THE TASTE

While some animals love the taste of coconut and will eat the oil "off the spoon," some don't take to it as easily. It is a new taste and some pets may hesitate to eat it or may refuse entirely. If your pet is trying coconut oil for the first time, give him just a little to try. He may turn his nose up at it at first and then come back later and give it a taste. "It was so funny!" says Gail speaking about her cat, "I put a tiny bit on my finger. She sniffed it for a bit, then put just the very tip of her tongue on it, and tasted it for a bit, then decided it tasted pretty good. When she was done, Atlas and Buster (her companions) licked her lips clean."

The best way to give coconut oil (or milk) to your pet is to combine it with food. It can be added to food in either solid or liquid form. For cats and dogs, about 1 teaspoon of oil for every 10 pounds of body weight has proven to be an effective daily dose. If your pet has a serious health issue, you may want to increase this amount until the problem is resolved.

Because coconut oil offers so many health benefits, it is worth giving it to your pet even if it has refused it earlier. If you mix it into their food, they may get used to the taste over time and begin to like it.

Izzy loves this stuff. I can pull it out and she sits pretty for it. Eats it straight off the spoon. Now my lab HATES it. I have to hide it in food or wrap cheese around it for her to even consider eating it. My favorite was when she ate the cheese and dropped the blob of coconut oil at Izzy's feet...We started out with 1/2 teaspoon and worked our way up to 2 tablespoons, one in the morning and one in the afternoon. Took us about two weeks to get there. Izzy would eat the whole jar if she had thumbs.
Anna

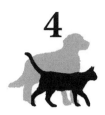

Skin, Hair, and Odor

Body odor, bad breath, dull coat, excessive shedding, and dry, flaky, irritated skin, claws, and hooves are all signs of poor health. One of the most noticeable effects of coconut oil reported by pet owners is improvement in their pet's skin, hair, and smell. Coats take on a silky, shinny, healthy luster and shed less. Body odor and kitty litter odor dramatically diminish. Bad breath becomes sweet. Bald spots, rashes, and other skin irritations go away. The pets look and feel healthier and happier.

Coconut oil improves the appearance of animals by improving their overall health. Coconut oil boosts immune efficiency, improves digestion, enhances nutrient absorption, aids in eliminating toxic waste, and kills bacteria and yeast that often contribute to foul smells and poor health.

Applied topically, coconut oil works wonders for just about any skin condition. I don't know of any other natural or commercial cream or lotion that can do so much for the skin and hair. It is good for treating dry flaky skin, cracked or irritated paw pads, chapped noses and flaky beaks, calloused elbows, irritated ears, hot spots, and rashes. It soothes irritated skin, clears up fungal and bacterial infections, and speeds the healing of cuts, wounds, bites and stings.

If your pet has a skin issue, massage coconut oil directly on the affected area and put additional oil in its food. Skin problems respond more quickly when the oil attacks the problem from both inside and out. For best results, apply the oil topically several times a day.

Here are a few comments from pet owners about the healing uses of coconut oil.

Our two cats love it. It has helped heal dry, flaky skin and coarse hair on one of them. His coat is now shiny and soft.
Kim E.

I'm no expert, but I can tell you every skin condition I have used the virgin coconut oil for, including my dogs very inflamed itchy skin, it has worked wonders on. It is very soothing to the skin. I think it would be beneficial since it has the antifungal, antiviral properties in it.
Valerie

We had a Pomeranian that gets hot spots every summer time and I use medicated ointment. Then, one summer I decided to experiment and use coconut oil instead and in less than 5 days, her hot spots went away.
Sheilah S.

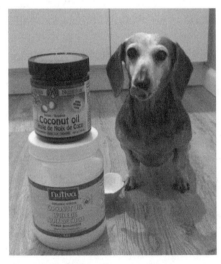

Cassie licks her lips as she waits patiently for her coconut treat.

I just put coconut oil on Maggie Mae (Poodle Bischon mix) for itchy skin, and she hasn't scratched since. Coconut oil to the rescue! She was licking it off my fingers and her skin, too.
Julianne B.

My dog and I both have a slice of whole grain bread smeared with coconut oil every morning. He can't wait for me to sit down and start eating, because he knows there's one waiting for him, too. I have to discourage him from wanting to give me a courtesy tongue bath when I use coconut oil as a moisturizer. He also loves coconut water. He's a true coconut aficionado. It does keep his coat shiny, helps his dermatitis, keeps his energy level up even here in Central America where it's a bit warm for a long haired golden retriever. Helps his shedding, maybe because there is less scratching, but I still think there's less shedding too. I read sometimes animals shed due to deficient diets.

B. B.

I have two German short hair pointers that are constantly shedding. If you pet them your hand ends up full of hair. My wife is constantly vacuuming hair everywhere. About 3 or 4 weeks ago I started feeding them a spoonful of coconut oil every day. Last night I was noticing how their coat shined and the shedding completely stopped.

Jack D.

My dogs LOVE coconut oil! One is quite overweight even though they all eat the same diet—including treats. Since starting it, their coats are glossy, more energy, and Cinnamon (handsome collie/chow mix) is actually losing some weight!...I started them on about a teaspoon each. Five of them get 1-2 teaspoons a day—just as a supplement—no health issues.

Debbie

I have three female Labradors. Usually when they are shedding at this time of year they will have a strong 'doggy' odor. The oldest dog has also had a chronic ear infection for years; the vet treats, it comes back, etc.

Six weeks ago I began giving the dogs each a heaping tablespoon of coconut oil per day, as well as wiping out the infected ear with melted coconut oil on a Kleenex. They adore the taste and will line up for their dose when they hear me open the jar.

I can now have all three dogs in the house and there is virtually no odor, and the ear infection has cleared up. In addition, their coats are beautiful. Normally it takes them a long time to get rid of all the dead winter coat, but this year the whole process was much faster.

They look so shiny and healthy! Also cleared up doggy breath.

Can't say enough good things about the effect of coconut oil on my dogs' health and well-being!

Patti

Belkie is a long haired Chihuahua mix and he was in very poor condition when we rescued him. You could feel every bone in his body, he had several bad teeth that needed pulling and his coat was very course. He cowered around and was very sad. After having him about a month and having some dental work done, his health and attitude improved. However, I still could not get him to stop itching. He did not have one flea on him, but he still itched! I added virgin coconut oil to his food and in no time he stopped itching and his coat is shiny, soft, and bright. He is the happiest little guy you ever saw!

S. F.

I thought that if coconut oil worked so well on humans, would it help my dog? We have been battling an unknown skin issue with my poor dog for almost two years. We tried a special diet. Antibiotics and medicated creams would help for a while and then the itch rash, redness, and lesions would return. I was so frustrated. So, I tried the oil on him daily and after three days I could see an improvement. In about two weeks, the skin was clear for the first time in two years! I shouted for joy and almost cried. My dog is not miserable anymore and neither am I. I apply the oil now about once a week. We all have some in the morning too.

Deborah W.

My two golden retrievers have been receiving 2-3 tablespoons of organic extra virgin coconut oil every single day for the past 4+ years. It is phenomenal for their digestion, skin, coat, etc. Our two consume a 100 percent grain-free diet (dry and raw foods), so the added bonus of coconut oil is a perfect complement to their nutritional regimens. I promote the use of organic extra virgin coconut oil to anyone who's interested in learning about its many benefits for canines. Providing canines with healthy doses of raw, unprocessed fats is the best type of food/supplementation you can give them. This is what their bodies are designed to eat, and the differences in their energy level, skin, and coat are highly noticeable...

For past clients whose dogs I've placed on coconut oil along with a healthy food regime, the documented results were astounding: significantly improved coat sheen and texture, quick hair growth around elbow calluses and areas of raw skin, less shedding, significantly reduced skin inflammation, healthy weight loss, and significantly improved energy.

Stella J. Raasch, BS,

Diplomat-Advanced Canine Nutritional Sciences

My 8 year old German Shepherd, Jojo, was chewing the base of her tail raw. She started doing it as the weather was changing to winter. A bald spot was developing, so I began massaging coconut oil all over her hind end. She couldn't get enough of the massaging while it was going on (a wonderful time of bonding), and got much relief afterwards. Her skin wasn't bothering her so there wasn't much chewing going on, she could lick herself afterwards safely, and the hair grew back in promptly.

Marty M.

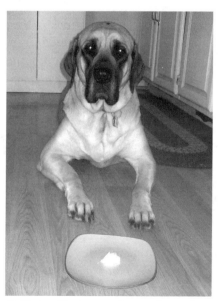

Bella's skin issues have cleared up since she began eating coconut oil.

It is that time again. Hot and muggy weather awakening the allergens and fleas! Bella, my dog, suffers from skin allergies. On top of this, she is prone to ear infections. When she arrived here, she began scratching her skin and digging her ear. She had an ear infection and skin allergies. The vet promptly put her on antibiotics and steroids. The steroids were to address the skin irritation. The antibiotics cleared her ear infection, but her skin continued to irritate her.

41

With her persistent scratching and discomfort from her skin, the vet suggested another round of steroids. Being hesitant to use more steroids, I opted to seek an alternative treatment. I found coconut oil for dogs is the alternative treatment I was searching for. It worked! Her skin began to clear and I saw her eyes light up. She felt great and loved the new treat, coconut oil!"

Kate

I put CocoTherapy on Pedro's paws as he has had issues before with cracking. Since we have been using it, no more cracks! His coat is also more shiny!

Gigi M.

I heard about it from my mom who is a "crazy cat lady" as she has 8 cats. She was tired of stepping in hairballs all day long, but didn't want to give her cats the hairball formula cat food from the vet, because of the by-products, grains, and chemicals in the food. She's been giving her cats both the oil and the coco chips for a few months, and since then, her cats have not barfed up hairballs in months!

She has been singing praises to CocoTherapy and telling everyone who has cats about it, so much so that I decided to try it for my cat (and my dog too). My cat's black and used to have white "dandruff" flakes on her skin and fur. Now the flakes are gone, and her fur shines like silk and feels like mink! My cat wasn't crazy about the chips, but I sprinkled it in her food, mixed with some water. Since eating the chips, she hasn't barfed a hairball in over 5 months! My dog loves the oil and chips too, he goes crazy for them.

Mary S.

Manny has greatly benefited from taking CocoTherapy daily. After just 3 weeks of taking the oil and chips, the bald spots on his chest and leg are starting to fill in with fur.

Now his leg hair has completely grown back! We had given up hope and had accepted the fact that we would have a dog with bald patches...and then we saw the CocoTherapy working its magic on his legs. His legs started out with sparse hairs here and there...and then after three weeks it started to look like it was filling in...and now he's back to his full leg hair. His chest hair is still growing in. It's taking longer than the rest because it's where his hair loss had begun first. But I definitely see progress! And he has stopped nibbling at himself and itching at himself.

Nikki F.

Have we personally seen benefits from adding coconut oil to our horse's diet? Yes! We first tried a coconut oil blend that was easy to pour on his grain, but when we ran out, we switched to virgin coconut oil. The only disadvantages I've found in using pure coconut oil have been a higher cost, and difficulty getting it out of the jar on a cold day.

Dollor's coat is shinier, his fur thicker, therefore his skin better protected and less sensitive. If minor skin issues come up, I sometimes rub the pure oil on him externally to cleanse and soothe. We've given him a hoof supplement for over a year, yet it wasn't until we added the coconut oil to his diet that his back hooves finally grew out with no splits.

The good results we saw with Dollor inspired us to put Sadie, our Great Dane, on a similar product called Coconut Cream Concentrate, which is 70 percent oil, combined with some coconut pulp. Sadie loves it so much that if I forget to add it to her food, she'll sit and stare sadly at the bowl until I remember! Her black coat is the shiniest it's ever been, and she often gets frisky, despite turning 8 years old! Last week her veterinarian marveled at Sadie's excellent health, amazed that she's the right weight and has no joint issues, either.

I can't prove coconut oil works, nor can I guarantee it'll meet your needs, but our happy horse and dog are proof it's working for us!

Cindy K.

OTHER SKIN ISSUES

Coconut oil is good for just about any type of skin condition—warts, moles, wounds, cuts, burns, sores, insect stings and bites, infections, and more. Coconut oil is anti-inflammatory, antibacterial, antifungal, and antiviral as well as a tissue knitter. It speeds the cellular repair processes in the skin, shortening the healing time. It makes an excellent topical healing lotion for all types of skin conditions.

My friend has a cat who had a round sore on his forehead that would not heal. I gave her a small tub of coconut oil with lavender oil that I used for my skin issues. She called me a few weeks later to let me know his sore was healed and that fur was growing back over the area. A couple of months later, she showed me that it was completely healed and I couldn't tell where the sore had been.
Patti T.

Our dogs love to eat it. My dog one day got a clean gash on his leg about an inch in size, I lashed on the coconut oil and bandaged it up to hold the cut together. When I brought him to the vet the next day it was hard to find the cut, it has healed together. She was amazed.
Shauna W.

Both my dogs love it. My lab's coat is like silk and shines like velvet. Coconut oil also helps remove warts and moles. I put some on my dog's wart daily and after several weeks it was gone.
Diane

A friend's cat got his tail caught in a door and she wasn't sure what to put on the wound (broken skin, bleeding, bruising) to keep it from getting infected. I had just read a description of coconut oil's topical use on serious cuts, and she happened to have some virgin coconut oil in her cupboard, so she applied it generously. The wound healed fast, even though the cat kept trying to lick the oil off.
C. J.

My pug, Piggie, had a weird rash that was in just one area on his belly. It was red and ugly. I didn't want him on meds and I didn't want to put meds on it for fear he would lick it. So I got my coconut oil and rubbed it on there. He would just lay there while I did it. Any other time he would squirm and try to get away. I think he liked the

smell of the coconut oil. He would, of course, lick it, so I would put more on him. And before bedtime I put more on. The red nasty rash started looking better and better every day. It finally was gone and you can't even tell where the rash was!
Cheryl W.

We use it for our Doxie who gets rashes on her belly. Cool bath then slather her belly in coco oil. No more itching!
Lindsay H.

We've seen many wonderful changes since we started using CocoTherapy oil and coconut chips. Shinier coats, weight loss—this works for us because they love the oil and chips and think they are "treats." I use it on their paws and no more dry, cracked paw pads! And last but definitely not least—no more straining for their poopies! We lovingly call it CocoMagic around our house.
Gina H.

BODY ODOR AND BAD BREATH

Does your dog's breath make your face cringe or your cat's liter box make your eyes water? If so, it's about time you do something about it. While pet odor is common, it isn't normal. It is a sign of ill health. Smells can be caused by poor diet, toxic buildup, allergies, skin infections, ear infections, tooth decay, gum disease, urinary tract infections, kidney disease, hypothyroidism, cancer, diabetes, ulcers, digestive disturbances, inflammatory bowel disease, immune system overload, or age-related changes. Often dogs smell bad because their bodies are constantly detoxifying the poor quality, unnatural ingredients found in many processed pet foods. Pet foods high in grains, soy, and other fillers are hard for them to digest.

Pet odor has become a major problem and treating this issue has developed into a booming business. A multitude of available products makes treating pet odors a complex and often confusing process. There are shampoos and soaps galore, steroids, antibiotics, dietary supplements, ear drops, toothpaste, breath fresheners, deodorizing sprays, and more. You have a choice of a dozen or so products to treat skin and hair odor, half a dozen or more products to treat bad breath, another half dozen for ear odor, more for gastrointestinal and anal odors, and still others for allergy caused odors. The list goes on and on. You almost have to have a PhD in odorology to treat all the possible causes of bad pet smells.

You could go broke buying all these products, not to mention all the time and energy you would need to spend putting them to use. None of these products, however, address the real problem—the health of your pet. They are temporary measures to control odor, not eliminate it or remove the underlying cause. Offensive odors are signs of health problems and should not be ignored or covered up.

One of the most enthusiastically welcomed results of using coconut oil is its remarkable deodorizing effects. There is no need for 52 different deodorizing products, one each for every imaginable source of odor. One simple inexpensive product can do it all for you.

Abby is our Labrador puppy. She smelled a bit "doggy" and had a few itches. She loves the coconut oil—I put a spoonful in my hand and she greedily laps it up, and I rub it on her coat. The doggy smell has disappeared, as have most of the itches. Her coat is glossy and beautiful.

M. A.

My Labrador puppy has the most beautiful black coat and no puppy smell. She loves the oil. Each morning she takes her place in the kitchen waiting for me to give her a spoonful in my hand, which she eagerly laps up. Even her favorite treats don't tempt her away from the oil.

M. R.

I have been feeding coconut oil to my husband's red tabby, Pumpkin. He was climbing into my lap at the table trying to steal it away, so I started putting half a teaspoon in his dinner. I have gradually increased the amount to 1 teaspoon. Almost immediately, we noticed a difference in odor—his cat box used to smell awful whenever he used it, and now there's no odor at all. His breath has improved as well.

C. J.

46

I have been giving CocoTherapy oil and chips to my dogs, Pebbles and Daisy. They used to have this funky odor, not really stinky, but a really distinct smell. I kinda like it, because I'm so used to it, but my friends and family think the dogs just stink. It's not just their breath or ears, but just an overall smell from their skin, and also their feet, almost like a "cheesy" smell, kinda like Doritos.

Since I started giving them the oil and chips, the odor has disappeared. My husband thinks I'm bathing them more, but I'm not, they just lost that funky smell. This stuff really works!!! Pebbles, Daisy and I give it 10 paws up!!!

Jennifer M.

Our 13-year-old lab has made a huge turnaround since we started him on CocoTherapy in December. He had a really bad smell and ears were not healthy. Now, he smells good, his breath is good, his ears are great and we can tell he has more energy. We are so happy with his progress. This is the only thing we have changed so it really works.

Susan S.

I just started using coconut oil for my dogs on the advice of a friend. I was a little skeptical but thought I'd give it a try. One of my boxers has the worst smelling breath I've ever smelled! We've tried treats, brushing, you name it...nothing worked.

After a little over a week of feeding coconut oil right from a spoon (they love it!), no more smelly breath!!! It's amazing! She's 6 years old now and a little white in the face. She's been slowing down lately too. Now she's up and playing while the other three are sleeping! Another of my boxers has very dirty ears. I could clean them every day and never keep up. Not to mention, it hurt her to have me clean them at times. Again, after about a week or so, not much in there to clean! I went a week without cleaning them too and they were wonderful and pain free! I love this stuff!!

Doreen M.

I have started using coconut oil for my two dogs about a month ago when I ran out of salmon oil for them...my daughter and I use it all the time....My dogs absolutely love it. Frazier actually eats the oil first at his meals. I give them about a tbsp full twice a day. I noticed right after two weeks that their coats got really soft, softer than with the salmon oil and shiny. I also read somewhere online that someone noticed that the "doggy" smell was gone. I wasn't sure that I believed this one but Frazier always had a "doggy" smell even a couple of days after his bath, but I have to say that when I started the oil he was starting to smell "doggy" and now after a month it's gone completely! He always smells so sweet now. I know it's crazy but it's true. I am going to keep using it.

Barbara

I regularly feed my pooches 1 tablespoon of coconut oil daily. I have a Springer and the breed is susceptible to allergies and ear infections. I have had the hardest time with these symptoms with him, and then the residual BAD, BAD, HORRIBLE breath from the oral bacteria that they also tend to hold. After dealing with numerous meds from the vets, I heard from Granny Good-Food that coconut oil would help in more ways than just the aforementioned. Sure enough, the coconut oil has completely cured the breath issue, and has helped tremendously with the allergy issues and ear infections.

Heather F.

SHAMPOOING AND TRIMMING

You can improve your pet's appearance by brushing or combing its coat every day to remove old hair or fur and debris that may be caught in it. Dead, flaky skin, oozing sores, pus, yeast and fungal infections, and body oil buildup mixed with dirt and debris can all contribute to offensive odors. Some pet odors are chemically bound to the skin and hair so that periodic shampooing is beneficial even though they are getting coconut oil on a regular basis. Make sure to wash out all the shampoo when you are done. Residual shampoo can also make your pet itch and smell. A good cleaning includes shampooing, rinsing thoroughly, and drying.

You can enhance the appearance of your pet's coat by using coconut oil as a hair conditioner. Rub coconut oil on your hands and then massage it into the animal's coat. You don't need to drench your pet in oil. Use just enough oil to apply a thin layer over the entire animal. It is best to do this outside so you don't get oil in your carpet and house. Let the oil soak in for 15 to 30 minutes. By this time much of the oil may have been licked off, but that's ok. Now wash your pet with soap and water as you normally would. You don't need to worry about getting all the oil out, just the excess. Much of the oil will be absorbed into the skin and hair. After the bath your pet's coat will take on a luxuriously healthy sheen.

Most oils do not absorb very well into the skin. If you put a dab of corn or soybean oil on your arm it will remain greasy all day long. Coconut oil doesn't do that. Because of the smaller size of the fatty acids, and because they are more water soluble than other fats, they absorb into the skin very quickly. If you apply a thin layer of coconut oil to you own skin, it will absorb in just a few minutes. The skin, however, can only absorb so much oil until it becomes saturated. If you put coconut oil on your skin and it is not absorbed in about 5 minutes, then you used too much. The same is true with animals. If you can put on a very thin layer that will absorb in just a few minutes, you won't need to bathe afterwards. Coconut oil treatment is a good way to prevent tangled hair and split and broken hair shafts.

I use it and completely recommend it. My gelding's (horse) tail is soft, shiny, and strong. Because it's so moisturized, there's no breakage of the hair, so his tail has gotten longer and thicker, since the hairs are having the chance to grow all the way down instead of just break off at his cannon bone…Coconut oil is the only oil that fully penetrates. It soaks in around 30 minutes or so, and doesn't leave a nasty feel afterwards. Just a soft tail…It doesn't take a whole lot, but in case you use a lot, it will still soak in completely, just over a longer period of time. You really can't use too much to the point of oiliness. The stuff soaks in fast.

N. G.

Sometimes it may be helpful to clip your pet's hair in order to access an infected or irritated area of skin and also perhaps alleviate odor that may be associated with it. This is especially true for long-haired cats infected with fungal ringworm. In addition to making it easier to treat and visualize problem areas, clipping makes it easier for affected skin to dry. Dry skin is more resistant to fungal, yeast, and bacterial infections than damp skin. Moist skin, especially in folds and creases, is prone to infections. Clipping makes shampooing and drying easier and the application of coconut oil or medications more effective and less messy.

The hair on most cats and dogs grows back quickly. Some cold weather dog breeds, such as Alaskan Malamutes and Siberian Huskies, grow and shed their coats only once a year or once every two years. When these dogs are clipped, their coats may remain short for many months.

A WORD ABOUT BIRDS

Parrots are among the most common of our feathered pets. There are many breeds; the small ones include parakeets, cockatiels, lovebirds, and lorikeets while the larger breeds include Amazons, African greys, cockatoos, and macaws. Common non-parrot birds include finches, canaries, doves, and pigeons, as well as outdoor birds like chickens, ducks, guinea hens, swans, and geese. Regardless of the type of bird you have, adding coconut and coconut oil to their feed can do them a lot of good.

The appearance of an animal can tell you a lot about its level of health. With mammals, you know there are health issues if they have a dull coat, itchy skin, flaky nails, or poor dental health. Likewise, you can tell the health of a bird by looking at its skin, feathers, beaks, and claws.

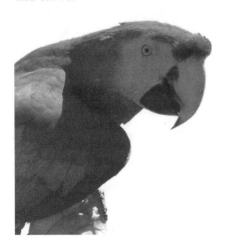

Diet plays a major role in the health of our pets. Over the years, bird feed has evolved and improved to include a mixture of seeds and grains along with fortified vegetable-based pellets. The pellets are customized to meet the nutritional needs of different types of birds, each breed receiving the food most suited for it. Fresh fruit and vegetables are recommended to round out the diet. This combination of food is believed to provide domesticated birds with all the nutrients they need for optimal health. Despite this scientific approach, birds often still suffer from certain diet related health and behavior problems, including the following:

- Dull feathers and poor pigmentation
- Excessive powder down
- Dry, flaky beak and claws
- Excessive grooming and self-mutilation
- Itchy, irritated skin
- Toe-tapping, wing-flapping, and feather-picking

It is apparent that there is something still missing in their diets, something birds in the wild appear to get that domesticated birds lack. Birds in the wild eat a more varied diet since they eat what nature provides rather than what pet food manufacturers deem suitable. One key nutrient that is sorely deficient in commercial bird food appears to be fat. In the wild, even vegetarian birds sometimes eat insects or have access to seeds and nuts that supply additional sources of fat. Our own fear of eating too much fat has spilled over into the formulation of pet foods. In addition, the fat that is in commercial bird food is probably old and rancid, which is not something that would promote good health. Like us, birds need essential fatty acids and fats in general for optimal health.

Dr. Karen Becker, a veterinarian who runs an avian hospital, was mystified by the fact that while birds seemed to receive a nutritionally sound diet, they still experienced the many health problems listed above. She suspected that fat was the missing nutrient in their diet and began supplementing her own birds. "I noticed several improvements," says Dr. Becker. "My African gray's dull tail, which also had a stress bar (a horizontal black line devoid of color or pigment), became a vibrant red color and the stress marks disappeared. My umbrella cockatoo's flaky beak and very dry feet improved. And my eclectus with the dull green feathers, some of which were actually black, returned to his wonderful bright green hue. I noticed a dramatic improvement not only in the condition and appearance of my flock's feathers, but also in their attitudes and behaviors. They were better able to focus, and in fact, my African gray's vocabulary began to expand."

The changes she noticed were enhanced with the addition of coconut oil. "When I started giving my flock coconut oil as their fatty acid supplement, the changes were dramatic. Three months after I added the oil to their diets, the condition of their feather coats was remarkably improved. Six months and a full molt later, they looked like different birds—so much so that I documented the changes in pictures. I also started recommending coconut oil to clients at my avian clinic."[1] Just as coconut oil improves skin and fur condition in mammals, it improves skin and feather condition in birds.

Never put oil of any type in a bird's water though; mix it into the food. One eighth teaspoon of coconut oil per day for every 1 pound (450 g) of body weight is a good amount, although you can give a little more without worry. Liquid (melted) coconut oil can be mixed into the feed. Birds generally love the taste of coconut oil and will eat it in its solid form. A pea size piece of hardened coconut oil per pound of body weight is about the same dose as the above. You can also feed them fresh or dried coconut meat. After all, coconut is just another type of seed and is readily eaten by birds in the wild. Read below what bird owners have said about their experiences with coconut and coconut oil.

I think these birds have a source of natural oil in the wild that we just don't realize. Some of the cockatoo varieties are open farmland plains type birds, but some of them like the U2, come from rain forest type areas. Kiwi has been given coconut, but I never thought to use some oil. I did increase (with vet consult) her increase of almonds this last winter. Just had a vet well-bird checkup and wing clip... Vet could hardly cut her wing feather shafts they were so strong. Vet commented how beautifully feathered she was and the strong feather shafts, and told me she is the best conditioned bird they've seen.
Janie

I use only the virgin coconut oil and I don't just give it to my flock straight. I use it in their birdie breads and sometimes mix a little into their chop mix. I use it in place of butter in recipes also, and since my birds eat a great deal of our foods they get it that way also.
Deborah

My Amazon has a dry, flaky, itchy beak. He is constantly rubbing his beak against his feet to scratch it. I've been using coconut oil lately to soften my skin after showing. It works for me, so I wondered if it would help with Charlie's beak. I gently began putting a little of the oil on his beak. It did the trick, his beak looks healthy and shiny and he's stopped scratching it on his feet.

B. W.

The other morning I awoke to lots of blood in TIKI's aviary (my Ducorps Cockatoo) evidently somehow she had cracked her beak quite seriously...unbeknownst to me....after bathing her because her feathers were quite bloody from her preening which I did not know at the time... I realized the blood was from her beak...The beak was seriously fractured AND still bleeding...of course it was the weekend with NO avian vets available....I was at a loss... So after cleaning TIKI, seeing she was calm...I took the coconut oil in my hands and abundantly on my fingers...TIKI rested her beak upon my fingers..... as if it were comforting...as if the bird KNEW this was going to help....for 15-20 minutes we continued applying more coconut oil and the bleeding subsided.....to BOTH our relief!!!!! Then, as I worried...I decided that it would be best to only offer TIKI soft foods and liquids with ALOE and coconut oil only, which TIKI nibbled at slowly but surely....each day TIKI healed remarkably...TODAY.... four days later...there is little evidence of TIKI's cracked beak... although I continue to feed TIKI oatmeal and veggies with coconut oil each morning very warmed and she eats very well.....So, I am convinced that the coconut oil indeed helped HEAL TIKI... TIKI is totally back to normal now.... I even had calls to several vets...who merely said IF I controlled the bleeding there was little they could do UNLESS infection set in...then antibiotics would be necessary... WELL.....thank goodness....COCONUT OIL IS INDEED antiviral and antibacterial....I BELIEVE this is TRUE now....with our specific situation....TIKI continues to rub her beak into coconut oil daily as if the bird KNOWS she NEEDS it!! NOW that is remarkable I THINK!!

Sandy

If you raise chickens, adding shredded coconut or coconut oil to their feed will improve egg production and egg quality. This

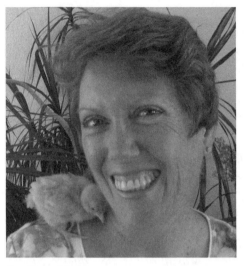
Leslie's chicks.

was revealed in a study published in the journal *Poultry Science*. The study lasted for 168 days and involved 200 chickens. The chickens fed the coconut grew larger during the study and were in better health, thus producing more eggs. It makes sense that healthy birds would be more productive than less healthy ones. Because of the antibiotic and antiviral properties of the oil, the chickens were probably less susceptible to infections and less vulnerable to salmonella and other potentially troublesome bacteria.

Coconut oil, but not coconut meal, also increased egg size. The amount of fat in the eggs

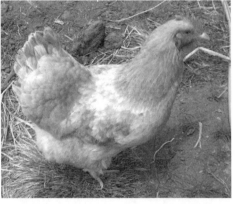

did not change but the type of fat did. Eggs from the coconut oil fed chickens had an increased amount of lauric acid, the primary medium chain fatty acid in coconut oil that gives the oil most of its health properties. The levels of stearic, oleic, and linoleic acids (long chain fatty acids) decreased.[2] In summary, adding coconut oil to the chicken feed improved the chickens' health, increased egg production and size, and improved egg quality.

5

A Natural Treatment for Infections

NATURE'S INFECTION FIGHTER

After nearly two months of intensive care, Aimee Copeland was released from the hospital to start rehab. Just a few weeks earlier she was on life support struggling to survive.

Aimee, a 24-year-old Georgia graduate student, was kayaking with friends when the accident happened. As a diversion, they decided to make a homemade zip line. An equipment malfunction on the zip line caused Aimee to fall and cut her leg. The injury was not that serious but it became infected with necrotizing fasciitis, commonly known as flesh-eating bacteria.

The infection spread quickly, eating away tissues throughout her body. Within days Aimee was battling for her life. She suffered with the failure of five major organs including her lungs and kidneys. To save her life doctors had to amputate her left leg, right foot, and both of her hands.

Necrotizing fasciitis is a severe bacterial infection that causes death in 1 out of every 3 cases. The infection is caused by so-called flesh-eating bacteria, spreading rapidly, destroying skin, muscles, and underlying tissues. The decaying flesh appears as if being eaten by the bacteria. The word "necrotizing" refers to something that causes body tissues to die. As the bacteria grow, toxins are released that kill tissues and interfere with blood flow to the infected area.

As the tissue dies, the bacteria enter the blood and rapidly spread throughout the body.

Treatment consists of broad-spectrum antibiotics given intravenously. Surgery is often needed to drain the sores and remove dead tissue. Skin grafts and amputation may be necessary if the disease spreads through an arm or leg.

There's no single kind of flesh-eating bacteria, many bacteria can be the cause. However, methicillin-resistant *Staphylococcus aureus* bacterium or MRSA causes a particularly nasty form of the disease because it is resistant to antibiotic therapy, making it very difficult to treat.

The medium chain fatty acids (MCFAs) in coconut oil possess potent antibacterial properties and are known to kill *Staphylococcus aureus* bacterium, including the drug resistant MRSA.

Can coconut oil be used effectively to treat bacterial infections? Many people have reported good results treating various infections in both themselves and their pets. In some cases, only coconut oil is used. In other cases, a combination of antibiotics and coconut oil has been successful. Clinical studies have shown that when used with conventional therapy, coconut oil can often speed recovery. Some of the most remarkable cases we hear about come from pet owners.

For example, the owner of Natural Pet Essentials related an incident that happened to one of her customers involving a Golden Retriever who had a recurring bacterial infection in his paw, and when they did a culture, they discovered that it was MRSA. Here is her story:

"In December 2011, my Golden Retriever was outside playing and cut the bottom of her paw. I was not aware of this until she began licking to heal what had already become infected. I took her to the veterinarian and he began her on a 28-day course of antibiotics. I cared for the paw by soaking it in Epsom salts 2-3 times a day and applying antibiotic cream and a clean dressing. When the course of antibiotics was complete, we still had an infected paw. She was again put on a 14-day course of medication. At that point, I was not seeing any response from the antibiotic so I consulted our veterinarian. He decided to take a culture of the area. It came back as MRSA! I was panicked. My option was one—to put her on the only known dose of antibiotic that would treat the infection. I was warned that this could be deadly (to the dog). I refused the treatment.

"I stopped in at Natural Pet Essentials, and I am sure glad I did. The knowledge that Kim had was incredible. She asked me to try coconut oil, since it is known to heal. I thought about it for all of one second and knew a natural remedy would be great if it would actually work. Let me just say: 'It worked!' I was amazed in as little as 3-4 days that her paw was looking much better and beginning to heal. The veterinarian was amazed also. I am now a permanent user of coconut oil and coconut chips for both of our dogs. Rylee, my Golden Retriever, is now a healthy and very happy 3-year-old Golden with a lot of spunk and willingness to play. If I had continued down the path of conventional veterinary medicine, I don't know if I would have my beautiful girl today. I am not saying that veterinary care is not good or important, I am just advising those with pets to look into other natural sources before giving in to [conventional veterinarian] medicine."

The MCFAs in coconut oil have been shown to kill a wide variety of potentially harmful bacteria, viruses, fungi, and parasites while remaining harmless to us and to our pets. In fact, our cells use MCFAs as food, absorbing these fatty acids and immediately converting them into energy. However, to tiny single-celled microorganisms, they can become deadly. Many of these organisms are encased in a fatty coat or membrane. Any cook knows that fat and water do not mix. Fats and oils, however, combine easily. This is how MCFAs kill germs. When MCFAs come into contact with microorganisms that have a fatty membrane, the MCFAs are easily absorbed into the membrane. Because of the fatty acid's small chemical structure, MCFAs weaken the organism's membrane, essentially dissolving it. The membrane splits open killing the organism. This is a process that bacteria cannot develop a resistance to, so MCFAs can kill the so-called superbugs, such as MRSA, that have become antibiotic resistant.

MCFAs can also kill viruses, including the flu virus and yeasts such as candida. Candida is a common inhabitant of the digestive tract in humans as well as pets. Therefore, it is easy for candida to find its way onto the skin, causing itching and skin rashes. Ears that are always dirty and inflamed, paws that smell like corn chips, and unpleasant body odor can all signal bacteria or yeast overgrowth.

When applied topically coconut oil can help get rid of skin infections. Taken internally it can help fight off systemic infections. Taken daily it can act somewhat like an inoculation that can help protect your pet from getting sick. While MCFAs can kill many troublesome microorganisms, it does not kill them all. You may need medications or other remedies to fight some infections.

In many cases, coconut oil works better than prescribed medications. "My dog has had furunculosis for years," says Beverly. Furunculosis is a recurring bacterial infection that is characterized by painful pus-filled boils on the skin, often occurring around the muzzle, anus, or toes. Relapses are common in affected dogs and they may be troubled by them for life. "Every autumn and winter when the ground is wet and muddy from rain and snow he gets furunculosis and has to be put on antibiotics," she says. "It gets better for awhile but in a week or two the problem is back." Beverly discovered that coconut oil had antibiotic and antiviral effects and that other pet owners had used it successfully to treat infections, so she decided to give it a try. "It only took about a week before the blisters started fading and in about two weeks he was completely healed. So far the furunculosis hasn't returned despite heavy raining and lots of mud and wet ground." Many other pet owners have experienced similar successes with other types of infections.

SKIN INFECTIONS

To treat skin infections, simply rub a little coconut oil on the infected spot. Your pet may lick it off so it is best to reapply the oil several times a day. You might also try adding clove oil, which possess very potent antimicrobial properties. Clove oil is very strong and can burn the skin so it must be diluted with another oil. Mix 2-3 drops of this essential oil into teaspoon of coconut oil. For a larger quantity, mix 30 drops (½ teaspoon) of clove oil with ¼ cup coconut oil. Do not apply clove oil directly to the skin as it is very strong and can cause blistering. It must be diluted with coconut oil before applying on the skin. Your pet may not like the taste of this mixture and in that case won't lick it off.

I am very pleased with the great benefits of coconut oil. My horse had these ugly warts on her nose that would not go away. I decided to put some coconut oil on them and everyone thought that I was going nutty. Within 6 days they had all cleared up and I am so

happy about it. She loves the smell and the taste of the oil too.
Tanya

We have a hairless Chinese Crested dog that developed skin lesions. I have no idea if they are bacterial, viral, or fungal. My understanding is that VCO has a broad spectrum of activity. Here are pictures (below) of the result of topical application of virgin coconut oil, starting with day 1 and the second picture is of day 7. We continue to apply virgin oil on her skin and we expect that the pigmentation will return soon.
Joey Testa

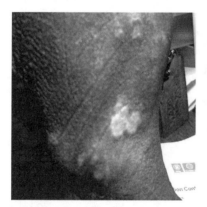 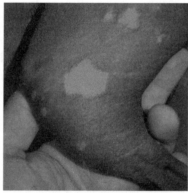

Hairless Chinese Crested dog before treatment (left), showing red, inflamed, and swollen sores. Seven days later (right) sores have healed leaving pink, smooth, healthy skin. The original dark skin pigment has not yet returned but the infection is gone.

Our dog had a small bump on his nose for about a month when I read the Whole Dog Journal article (about coconut oil) and it made me curious. The vet had said that it didn't look like anything to be concerned about, perhaps the result of a virus that he may have picked up from another dog or an insect bite. I checked around a bit and talked to a co-worker that's into health foods and decided to give the coconut oil a try. I put a dab on his bump once a day and in three days it was gone.
Anonymous

My rabbits had some kind of skin infection and my vet suggested applying coconut oil the infected areas. The coconut oil cleared the infection in just a couple of days, but I had to keep applying more coconut oil because they loved the smell and taste of it so much they would immediately lick it off.

K. D.

My dog Katie had a tiny pink lump on her chin. It gradually grew larger so we brought her to the vet, who diagnosed it as folliculitis (a skin infection surrounding hair follicles). He said to wait until it got bigger and he would do surgery to remove it. It grew to the size of a pea and became a very angry reddish pink in color. It was really terrible to look at and right on her pretty face! I didn't want to put her through the surgery so I decided to try coconut oil after reading about other's success with skin problems.

I applied coconut oil daily. Gradually the lump reduced in size and the color became normal. After about two weeks I noticed it had broken and become crusty. I kept applying the oil daily and now a month later it is very tiny and a normal skin color. I really had to look to find it! I'm really happy with the coconut oil.

Bernadette

I can't believe how quickly coconut oil heals skin problems caused by Valley Fever (fungal infection). Even dogs that are infected with this fungus respond well with this treatment.

M. M.

When my cat was sick, the ONLY thing that helped him was coconut oil. Nothing seemed to stop him from vomiting. Giving him a teaspoon of coconut oil a day stopped him from vomiting and he has gained his weight back. My cat is 16 years old and going strong now.

There should be no difference between an animal taking coconut oil versus a human. My dog loves the stuff, and she had such a pretty coat.

Penny W.

I have a goat that got a viral infection on her udder known as "goat pox." It is a type of herpes simplex virus. I later noticed

I had a little pustule on my wrist, in spite of my best efforts to use preventive sanitation while milking her. I put a dab of coconut oil on it, and it was gone by morning. A few days later there was another tiny pustule on my hand. I did the same thing with the same results. I treated the goat's udder with the coconut oil with good results.
Jill

After reading an article about coconut oil in a dog journal (The Whole Dog Journal), I decided to start giving my Rottweiler coconut oil when he developed what my vet described as warts, on his head. I put some of the oil on it two times a day and it just fell off after a couple of weeks. He got another one on his head months later in a different spot (had I left them they would have looked like little devil horns). I used the oil again, it fell off.
Angie C.

My eight-year-old English bulldog has pretty severe allergies and gets these "interdigital cysts" on occasion. She has taken a weekly shot concocted by her veterinarian dermatologist for four years...I put her on that four months ago. Last month, I took her off the shots. We have had a terrible pollen season this year in SE Texas, yet she has done fine on 2 tablespoons of CocoTherapy oil per day-- and no interdigital cysts.
Jay K.

Coconut oil is not limited to just topical applications, it can be added to the animal's food where it can work its healing magic throughout the body. In fact, for skin problems, applying the oil on the skin as well as eating it enhances recovery time.

I have a 14 year old Lhaso. For about two years now, she's had a scabby rash and all she did was lick it and itch 24-7. I was at my wits end with her, as I tried everything and she still itched. Well, this time last week I thought, what the heck if it's good for people then it'll be good for my dog Candy. So I put it in her food daily and rubbed it on that spot. It is totally unbelievable but Candy isn't itching and the spot seems to be going away.
P. S.

We rescued a young cat who we found at the park. Her eyes were full of gunk, her nose was sealed shut with snot. She sneezed and coughed constantly. We took her to the vet who told us she had a bad respiratory infection. She gave us traditional meds and we did them as we were told but with no improvement. This happened three times. Expensive! And poor Ali still was terrible and hated the meds. I knew that coconut oil had antibiotic properties, so I decided after the third round to try it. She loved the coco oil and within a week of giving her a small spoonful a couple times a day the snot and gunk were gone and she was no longer sneezing and coughing. We were thrilled and amazed! I wish we'd tried it to begin with! A few months ago we found another stray and he's got parasites. Coco oil once again and he's a new cat!

Lindsay H.

My dog developed sores just above his upper lip. The vet gave him an antibiotic, but it didn't seem to do any good. After a week I stopped the medication and began applying coconut oil to the sores. They got worse for a few days and then began to heal. He recovered without a problem.

L. J.

EAR INFECTIONS

Ear infections are common. Symptoms include itching (evidenced by digging at the ear), bad odor, shaking or tilting of the animal's head, and heavy discharge. Moisture trapped in the ear or frequent exposure to moisture creates a warm moist environment conducive to bacterial and fungal growth. The ear canal can be blocked and moisture trapped by ear wax buildup, dirt, dust, grass particles, and other debris. Mites and bugs may also find it to be a suitable home. Yeast is very common in ear canals and can be virtually impossible to eliminate completely. It can only be controlled by regular cleaning. Itchy scabs are common signs of yeast infections.

To treat an ear infection, first wash the ear with a damp cloth and a little soap. Try not to get any water down the ear canal. Using a cotton swab or ball of cotton, apply hydrogen peroxide to the infected area to kill the infection. It is all right if some of the hydrogen peroxide dribbles down the ear canal, it will just kill more microbes. Let the ear dry, then apply a thin coat of coconut oil. It's okay, too, to get some of the coconut oil into the ear canal. It is not harmful and can be beneficial.

If there is a lot of wax buildup, coconut oil can be used to dissolve and remove it. Use an eye dropper and put several drops of melted (but not hot) coconut oil into the ear canal. The oil will loosen up the wax, allowing it to drain from the ear naturally. Coconut oil in the ear canal will also help to control deep infections. This method can be used to treat active infections and, if used periodically, to prevent recurring infections.

My dog had very infected ears complete with swelling and the smell of infection. I started putting the coconut oil right in his ears and within a few days they were greatly improved. His ears are completely healed now.

V. A.

My dog has had a scabby, itchy spot on his ear for months. The vet said it's an allergy and gave me some lotion. The lotion never helped. The poor dog was suffering with this itchy scab, so on Tuesday I put coconut oil on it. I did that twice a day for two more days. Today is Friday and the scab is completely gone and the itchy patch is nearly gone! I am truly amazed.

M. T.

My female English bulldog has scabbed and crusty inside ear folds. I read on Facebook on a bulldog rescue that people had great results using this product (coconut oil) so I ordered some...After two applications her ears are completely healed up...Ever since finding this product she no longer gets ear infections or dried crusty ear folds. I even went as far as putting it on my hands, which use to get dried out every winter and crack and peel. I am pleased to say my hands are dry no more.

Wendi R.

EYE INFECTIONS

For infected or irritated eyes, coconut oil can work wonders. Coconut oil in the eyes? Yes, it is perfectly safe. Put melted coconut oil in an eye dropper and squeeze a few drops in each eye. There is no stinging, burning or irritation. I often do it to myself. When my eyes become irritated with dust or debris or when I think there may be an infection, the first thing I do is squirt in a few drops of coconut oil. It works with pets as well.

My dog is white and had terrible red tear stains on the corners of her eyes that went beyond her cheeks. I was afraid to try Angel Eyes because I heard it contained antibiotics. My vet recommended that I give her CocoTherapy coconut oil, as it has antifungal, antibacterial, antiviral, and anti-yeast properties. I'm thrilled because not only have the red stains on her eyes cleared up, the red stains on her paws, from her chewing them, have cleared up too!
Kris O.

Coconut oil is helping tremendously! It really is amazing. In just two days there is such a big difference. It is working ten times faster than the other remedies I was trying and with much better results. I'm also using it in all three of the dogs' food and I rubbed it in-between the pads of their paws and on their eyelids and no more redness or itching!
Sarah S.

ORAL HEALTH

Dental disease is the most common infection in dogs and cats. Almost all dogs encounter some dental problems by the age of three and 95 percent of all dogs and cats will experience some degree of dental disease in their lifetime.

As with humans, dental disease in animals starts when food particles accumulate in between and on their teeth. Bacteria in the mouth that eat these particles produce acids that weaken the teeth and make them susceptible to infection and decay. Some bacteria form colonies that coat the teeth, creating a sticky yellow film called plaque. If the plaque becomes calcified, it hardens into tartar. If enough plaque builds up it can cause infection of the gums. This is called gingivitis and is often seen as a red line (inflammation) along the junction of the teeth and gums. If the infection penetrates deeper into the gums it causes periodontal disease, which can lead to the loss of infected teeth and even affect underlying bone.

Eating hard foods or chewing on bones or other hard objects helps to scrape plaque off the teeth and stimulate saliva flow, which can wash trapped food particles away from the teeth. In dogs and cats the foods most prone to cause decay are carbohydrates—candy, dried fruit, grains, and starchy vegetables. Carbohydrates are broken down by salivary enzymes into sugar, which bacteria feed on. The more sugar available, the faster bacteria multiply and the more acidic the mouth becomes, weakening the teeth and making them more susceptible to infection and decay. Foods high in carbohydrate increase the risk of dental disease. Unfortunately, carbohydrate-rich ingredients make up a substantial part of many dog and cat foods. Corn, soy, and wheat, which are used as fillers in pet foods, are very high in carbohydrate.

Dirty teeth may look and smell bad, but the real damage is far worse. Gum tissue has an extensive blood supply. When periodontal infection sets in, oral bacteria can seep into the bloodstream. This bacteria is carried throughout the pet's body where it can infect any and every tissue and organ including the heart, kidneys, brain, and bone and joint tissues, causing secondary infections and even organ failure. Many cases of arthritis and heart and kidney failure have been traced back to oral infections. With a load of bacteria constantly seeping into the bloodstream, the immune system is under a heavy burden, resulting in low energy levels and frequent infections. Even cancer risk increases because the immune system is chronically depressed.

Symptoms of oral infections include bad breath, discolored teeth, inflammation (red gums), bleeding gums, tartar buildup, and sensitive teeth. In some cases, dental work may be necessary. However, feeding your dog or cat a healthy, low-carbohydrate diet along with adequate coconut oil can work wonders at improving oral health. Gum disease can reverse itself and even minor cavities are healed. Some people brush their pet's teeth using a canine or feline toothbrush and coconut oil mixed with a little baking soda. The baking soda is useful because it helps neutralize excess acids and balance pH in the mouth. Pet supply stores sell gauze wipes containing tooth-cleaning chemicals. You can make your own by wrapping your finger with gauze and dipping it in coconut oil and baking soda.

Signs of Severe Gum Disease
- Problems picking up food
- Bleeding or red gums
- Loose teeth
- Blood in the water bowl or on chew toys
- Bad breath (halitosis)
- Making noises when eating or yawning
- Bumps or lumps in the mouth
- Bloody or ropey saliva
- Not wanting the head touched (head shyness)
- Chewing on one side of the mouth
- Sneezing or nasal discharge (advanced gum disease in the upper teeth can destroy the bone between the nasal and oral cavity)

Fortunately a proper diet along with the addition of coconut oil can do wonders for your pet's oral health.

I give my dogs about a tablespoon a day and about 4 months after I started to do this, I noticed my dog's teeth were getting much whiter and their gums looked so healthy. They did have some build up prior to the coconut oil and that is now all gone except for a little on a couple of their far back molars, but I can see

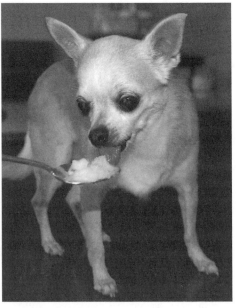

Coconut oil helps keep teeth and gums clean and healthy.

more and more white on those molars coming through all the time. I don't brush their teeth or do anything else for their teeth other than give them the coconut oil. Plus, their fur is very soft and extremely shiny.

Also, I have a cat that is 14½ years old now and he decided that he also likes coconut oil. As you can imagine, in a 14-year-old cat, his teeth were not the best. After about 2 months eating coconut oil (which he absolutely loves and will bug me to no end until I give it to him in the morning) I was looking at his teeth and they look amazing—white and pink healthy gums. Plus his energy has definitely increased. He is much more mobile and alert, and playful.

S. K.

Every night I rub some VCO on my dogs' teeth and they don't have bad breath anymore. Their coats are glistening.

Bonnie C.

I have two shelties, one of which has been missing six adult teeth since he grew in his adult teeth as a puppy. I've been giving my shelties coconut oil for nine months now and have noticed many benefits, such as a very silky coat and the plaque on their teeth has all but disappeared. Plus, their teeth are very white like they just had a cleaning, which I know I can credit to the coconut oil because I have read this before. But I'm amazed at my 3½-year-old sheltie growing in his missing teeth. He has three new teeth and I can see another one peeking through the gum line. I'm thinking it's the coconut oil balancing something in his system.

Ellen

My cat was diagnosed last year with gingivo-stomata-titis or something like that, the vet said it so fast, a progressive disease of the gums which would necessitate pulling all of her teeth (she was 3 at the time).

I started smoothing coconut oil on her gums every morning. She hates it, but hasn't figured out how to effectively hide from me. We went to the vet on Saturday, and he said he saw no evidence of the disease. I told him about the oil, and he said, "Hey, if it works, great?" But then he said he couldn't recommend it because he doesn't have scientific evidence for it. (And probably somebody would sue him if it didn't work).

Also, Princess' coat is thick, full, and oh so soft and her weight has actually gone down from last year. So don't be afraid to use coconut oil on your pets.

Laurie

Contrary to the position taken by the dentist in the story above, there are actually a lot of studies that demonstrate the antibacterial effects of the medium chain fatty acids in coconut oil. In a recent study by investigators from the Athlone Institute of Technology in Ireland, coconut oil was found to be very effective in killing bacteria that cause dental disease.[1] The research team tested the antibacterial action of coconut oil against various strains of Streptococcus bacteria, common inhabitants of the mouth. What they discovered was that the MCFAs in the coconut oil strongly inhibited the growth of most strains of Streptococcus bacteria including *Streptococcus mutans*—an acid–producing bacterium that is the primary causative agent of dental cavities. It was no surprise to other researchers in the field, since earlier studies produced similar results.[2]

6

Fleas, Ticks, and Other Parasites

PARASITIC PESTS

Summer is a perfect time for our furry friends to play outside. They love to roll around and romp through tall grass, explore new territory, and even chase other little critters about. Unfortunately, they often bring home some unwelcome guests—fleas, ticks, mites, lice, and other parasites.

These pests are a terrible nuisance to pets and humans alike. They reproduce quickly, are difficult to control, and can transmit parasitic worms and diseases that are dangerous to animals and humans. These little buggers can inflict humans with tapeworms, bubonic plague, typhus, cat scratch fever, Lyme disease, Erlichiosis, Rocky Mountain spotted fever, flea-borne spotted fever, tick bite fever, and meningoencephalitis—a viral infection that affects the brain and spinal cord.

Some of these tiny pests, primarily fleas, can cause parasitic dermatitis—an allergic reaction triggered by a hypersensitivity to substances in the fleas' saliva causing itchy, inflamed skin, and papules. Eventually the irritation may cause hair loss and bacterial infections. These symptoms can exist long after the flea infestation has been eliminated.

Fleas and Ticks

Pet owners are encouraged to use flea and tick protection products such as Frontline and Advantage II. We are instructed to apply these products to our pets every one to two months for complete protection. The active ingredient in these products is fipronil—a broad spectrum insecticide. Fipronil is used in a wide variety of products to kill ants, cockroaches, termites, and weevils, as well as fleas and ticks, and works by disrupting an insect's nervous system. When fipronil is applied, it spreads from the point of application across the animal's skin, taking about 24 hours to cover the pet's entire body. Fleas and ticks are killed on contact. Fipronil is absorbed into the pet's skin, hair, and sebaceous (oil) glands, maintaining protection for about four weeks. Of course, since it is absorbed into the skin, some of it will also end up in the pet's bloodstream. Possible side effects include drooling, skin discoloration and irritation, itching, hair loss, and vomiting. What else would you expect when poisons get in the body? Since fipronil is designed to disrupt nerve function in insects, it is also an environmental hazard and can kill wildlife—bees, birds, fish, etc. Continued use over time can cause nerve damage to pets.

Your choice is to either slowly poison your pet with these products, which might lead to serious disease later on, or let them suffer with the irritating infestation, struggle with allergic reactions, and risk possible transmission of disease from them to you. Is there a better option? You bet there is. You can get rid of fleas and ticks without harm to you or your pet. The solution is coconut oil.

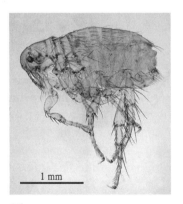

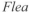
1 mm

Flea

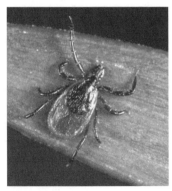

Tick

One parasitic insect that often torments humans as well as animals is the louse (singular for lice). Lice are small, wingless insects that feed on dead skin or blood. The lice that infect humans make their home on the scalp and other hairy areas, feeding on our blood. In many ways they are similar to the fleas, ticks, and mites that plague our pets. Coconut oil is a traditional folk remedy for lice. A generous amount of oil is massaged into the hair and allowed to sit for 8 to 12 hours. The oil is then washed out and along with it come all the dead lice. Coconut oil kills lice in a different manner than it does bacteria and other single-celled organisms. With lice, it is believed that the oil coats the exoskeleton of the pests, blocking off their oxygen, suffocating them. In addition to suffocating the parasites, the oil prevents bites and sores from becoming infected (due to its antimicrobial properties) and stimulates cell turnover and rapid healing (from its energy inducing and metabolic stimulating properties). These are things other oils cannot do. This same process should also work on other similar parasitic insects that torment our pets. According to the testimonies of many pet owners, coconut oil not only kills these little parasites but also keeps them away like an insect repellent.

I was concerned about the toxic effects of flea and tick medications so I went online to find a safer, natural solution. In my search I came across a variety of natural insect repellents such as eating garlic and applying essential oils like eucalyptus and neem. But most of these remedies have drawbacks too. The smell from these products can be unpleasant for both humans and pets and in some cases the oils can irritate the skin. One of the sites mentioned the use of coconut oil. Coconut oil has a mild, pleasant smell, is much cheaper than essential oils, is easier to get, and has no harmful effects. It was worth a try. I applied the oil to my dog's coat every time we went for a walk. Boy did it make her coat shine! She hasn't had any ticks or fleas since I've been using coconut oil. It gives better results than the commercial products I used to use and it's cheaper!
R. J.

Apply virgin coconut oil on the skin and rub gently on sores and flea bites. It works wonders and in a few days the sores and fleas are gone. The dog smells good too.
A. G.

Like me, my dogs get 1 ml per kg bodyweight (or more) every day and they love it. They will enthusiastically lick up any spills (and lick me too when I use virgin coconut oil as first aid on scratches and insect bites).

We live in an area (tropical north Queensland, Australia) with many dangerous ticks including the so-called 'paralysis tick' which kills many dogs and cats every year. Since starting my dogs on virgin coconut oil I have not found any ticks on them and they have no fleas either.

No need for any highly toxic (and expensive) chemical flea and tick control for my dogs.

Clemens V.

Scabies Mite

Unlike fleas, mites are not insects; they are arachnids and belong to the same family as spiders, and scorpions. The most distinguishing feature separating insects and arachnids is the number of legs. Adult insects have six legs, but mature mites, as well as spiders, have eight.

Sarcoptes scabiei, commonly known as the scabies, mange, or itch mite, is a parasite of humans and animals. The term *mange* is used to describe the poor condition of an animal's skin and coat due to a severe mite infestation.

Scabies mites are microscopically small, but sometimes may be visible as pinpoint sized specks of white. Scabies mites are highly contagious and are transmitted primarily by direct contact and through contaminated grooming equipment and kennels.

Pregnant female mites tunnel into the outermost layer of a host's skin where they feed on tissue fluids and deposit their eggs. Males roam on top of skin, only occasionally burrowing into the skin. In their burrows, females lay up to three eggs per day for a period of eight weeks, producing about 200 eggs over her lifetime.

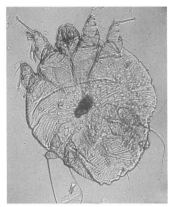

Scabies mite

These eggs hatch in three to ten days and the newly-hatched larvae emerge from the burrow onto the surface of the skin and molt into nymphs. The rash and intense itching associated with scabies occurs when the nymphs burrow into the skin and begin feeding. These symptoms usually appear a few weeks after the initial infestation. The life cycle, from egg to adult, can be completed in about two weeks. As soon as the female nymphs become adults, they begin to lay eggs.

Probably no other skin disease will cause your dog or cat to scratch and bite itself with greater intensity. Scabies mites commonly attack the skin of the ears, elbows, upper hind legs, and the underside of the chest and face. The onset of infestation is abrupt and marked by scratching, hair loss, and inflamed skin. Typically you will see thick gray to yellow crusts around the edge and tips of the ears. A classic test for scabies in dogs is to rub the ear flap between your fingers and watch the dog scratch on the same side. The same test would probably work for cats as well. In the later stages, the skin becomes thick, crusted, scaly, and darkly pigmented. Intense scratching can cause wounds that can become infected.

Conventional treatment consists of clipping off long hair around infected areas and bathing the entire animal with a benzoyl peroxide shampoo. The shampoo loosens the scales and crusts and makes it possible for an insecticide dip to penetrate deeper in to the pores and hair follicles. Scabies mites have developed resistance to a number of insecticide dips, so you would have to use a dip recommended by your veterinarian and dip the animal about once a week for eight weeks. Or you could use coconut oil and avoid the chemicals altogether.

I recently rescued a little Mountain Feist (small squirrel hunting dog) that had sarcoptic mange and skin infections. She had very little hair on her little body. She was treated for the mange and skin infection. I started giving her a teaspoon of coconut oil on her food every day. (Funny, she didn't like it at first but now she hunts it out and gobbles it down.) It's been about two months and her fur is beautiful, thick and glossy. I have two other dogs that I have NOT been giving coconut oil. All of the dogs have Advantix because the tick population is HORRIBLE in our area. What I have noticed is that with our daily hikes into the woods around us, my big dogs come back loaded with ticks (I'm talking 20 plus each) and the little one will usually have just one or two, if any at all. She runs through the woods in the same area as the other dogs, plus with her small size brushes her whole body against the grasses and bushes, and she will have no ticks! Is it the coconut oil? I am just really baffled as to why one dog out of three will not have any ticks.

Cassandra

You might be interested to know what really got my attention about coconut oil. We adopt guinea pigs and a few months ago our latest rescue, a beautiful black Peruvian, brought uninvited guests with her—mites! This is something we've never experienced before. I didn't know what was wrong but all five piggies were quickly going downhill, so I called Fenella (the founder of Wee Companions rescue) and she came by and treated them for mites. Everyone got a shot, then ivermectin (a drug used to treat parasite infections) once a week for three weeks. Their skin was awful and they almost itched themselves to death—literally. One actually had a seizure and was lifeless in my hands. I thought we'd lost her. Fortunately, I was able to bring her back by massaging her. However, after four weeks of meds, we still weren't over the problem. Their skin was crusty, they were quickly going bald, and they were biting holes in their skin and itching up a storm. When Fenella was here to doctor them, she agreed that there were a couple that were on their last legs—major crisis.

I did some research and found that Bag Balm was used successfully on piggies with mites, however, when I looked at the ingredients, I couldn't imagine putting that stuff on them, especially since they will often lick their fur when cleaning themselves. So, I decided to slather them with coconut oil for a couple of weeks. Twice a day I rubbed coconut oil all over each one of them. They were little grease fur balls with legs, but didn't seem to mind at all. I'm thrilled to report absolutely amazing results! In less than two weeks the mites were completely gone. Their fur is so thick and gorgeous, their skin looks great, they've got their energy back, and all five of them are the picture of health. In fact, they could easily be poster piggies for

the miracles of coconut oil. If I'd just done the coconut oil in the first place, they'd been well so much sooner—live and learn.
Kaye H.

I started using organic virgin coconut oil with a foster dog that had recently been treated for sarcoptic mange, and yeast and bacterial infections. The transformation of her skin and coat was amazing! I also started feeding it to my fosters who came to rescue with lesions and hair loss from flea dermatitis.

After seeing the difference VCO makes, I feed it on a regular basis to my resident dogs as well as my fosters. When my 6-year-old papillon/poodle mix had her last checkup, her vet was extremely complimentary about the condition of her coat.
Caryn F.

I had a great experience of the medical magic of coconut oil. Last month I was rearing a kitten which was suffering from a skin disease called scabies. I took it to the vet and he gave me medicine named RID. I was washing the kitten with that medicine mixed in water, but no result came and the kitten died from the disease.

This month I rescued another kitten abandoned by her mother. This kitten also started showing symptoms of scabies. As I had a bad experience with the doctor in the last case, my mom decided to do her own treatment with the kitten at home. My mom spread coconut oil on the cat's body where it was infected by scabies. She did this daily, once a day. You won't believe it, but the kitten recovered from that disease and is now playing with lots of energy.
Palak T.

INSECT REPELLENT AND HEALING SALVE

Coconut oil has often been used as an insect repellent. I use it as a sun block when I spend any time outdoors in the sun. I often visit tropical locations where mosquitoes, sand flies, and other annoying insects abound and have noticed that when I don't put on coconut oil, I end up with many insect bites. When I do rub it onto my skin, the bites are minimal and if I do get bitten, the pain and itching is far less severe. If I do get bitten or stung, coconut oil takes away the irritation and inflammation and speeds healing.

I discovered your book The Coconut Oil Miracle *while searching for a fly spray for my horse. He has a hyperactive immune system and the natural sprays with essential oils gave him hives. Our vet said she had just heard about using coconut oil as a fly spray for cows producing organic milk. I immediately headed to the natural market and came home with your book, a gallon of organic coconut oil for my horses, and a jar of virgin coconut oil for me. It works!*
Debbie W.

I feed my dog a tablespoon of virgin coconut oil every morning and I put some in her food. She loves it and her coat is shiny. The other day she got stung by a bee and her mouth was swollen. I rubbed some virgin coconut oil plus gave her a tablespoon and within an hour the swelling had gone down and she was up and about.
Michelle

INTESTINAL PARASITES

There are two general groups of intestinal parasites. One consists of worms such as tapeworms and roundworms. The second category is made up of protozoa, or single-celled organisms. Parasites infect the intestines of both humans and animals and can cause a great deal of intestinal distress.

Parasites are a continual threat to animals, especially if the animals are outdoors a lot. Giardia and cryptosporidium are the most common single-celled parasites. They normally live in the digestive tract of animals and are spread though fecal contamination. Most surface water is contaminated with these organisms and uninfected animals become infected from drinking out of lakes, streams, and ponds. Symptoms may range from mild, recurring diarrhea consisting of soft, light-colored stools, to acute, explosive diarrhea in severe cases. Other signs include weight loss, listlessness, fatigue, and mucus or small amounts of blood in the feces.

It is believed that 5 to 10 percent of all dogs in North America are infected with giardia at any given time. Surveys show that over 30 percent of dogs under one year of age have been infected at some point during their life. Another study found that 100 percent of the kennel dogs studied, 50 percent of the pups, and 10 percent of the well-cared for dogs carried giardia. Healthy animals can fight off the infection but in those with a weakened immune system or those who are repeatedly exposed to the parasite, the infection can become chronic. Drugs are available for treating this parasite but the side effects can be severe.

Intestinal worms are a fact of life for dogs and cats, and even puppies and kittens can be infected. Pets should be dewormed regularly, whether or not an infection is suspected. The most common worms that infect our pets are roundworms, tapeworms, whipworms and hookworms. Pets can pick up worms from their mother during birth, by ingesting parasite eggs, or through a bite from an intermediate host, such as a mosquito or tick.

A number of natural dewormers have been suggested such as a 24 hour fast followed by a high-fiber diet or eating certain foods or supplements like raw garlic (not recommended), crushed pumpkin seeds, wheat germ oil, digestive enzymes, and various herbs. Natural dewormers are often ineffective and sometimes harmful. Some natural methods such as digestive enzymes are better used as preventatives and may not affect all the different types of parasites that could infect your pet. Over-the-counter dewormers are generally not very effective and can be toxic. Prescription wormers are a more effective treatment but they can be harsh and produce unpleasant side effects.

Coconut has long been used in the coconut growing regions of India as a treatment for intestinal worms in humans. Whenever someone was infected with parasites, the traditional remedy was to

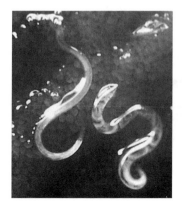 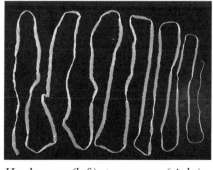

Hookworm (left), tapeworm (right).

eat large quantities of coconut meat. This was reported to kill or expel all the worms living in the digestive tract. After many generations of use, researchers in India finally decided to put this old "wives' tale" to the test and evaluate its effectiveness under strict scientific conditions.

The investigators went to a village in India where tapeworm infestation was epidemic. Fifty infected individuals volunteered for the study. The subjects were given either fresh or dried coconut to eat along with a laxative to assist in the expulsion. They found that coconut did indeed expel the tapeworms and that dried coconut was twice as effective as fresh coconut. Those consuming dried coconut expelled 90 percent of the parasites within 12 hours.

Not only did the dried coconut work, but it was more effective than most anti-parasitic drugs used for this purpose and about as effective as Niclosomide, the most popular and potent anti-tapeworm medication. Niclosomide works by causing tapeworms to

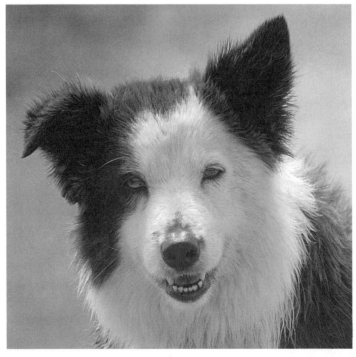

A parasite-free pet is a happy pet.

waste away in the patient's digestive tract, which releases toxins that can cause undesirable side effects. Coconut, on the other hand, is completely nontoxic, palatable, and available without a prescription.

Dried coconut (which would include coconut chips and desiccated coconut), and to a somewhat lesser extent fresh coconut, can help prevent and expel worms in humans. You might assume that it would also work in similar ways in animals. This, in fact, is the case. Not only is coconut meat an effective dewormer but so is coconut oil. The first time I heard of coconut oil being used for this purpose was from a woman who called me and excitedly exclaimed that when she started giving her cat coconut oil, it began passing worms in its stools. After three days, no more worms. The cat was worm-free. She was thrilled to find a natural, palatable solution to this problem. Perhaps a combination of both dried coconut and coconut oil mixed with food would be the best natural treatment for worms.

Coconut oil has an added benefit over other natural and prescription dewormers; it also kills single-celled parasites such as giardia and ciliate protozoa that may also infect an animal's digestive tract. This has been verified by medical research. The regular addition of coconut oil to your pet's food can help to keep both types of intestinal parasite infections at bay.

My cat is an addict...he acts like it is cat nip...it makes him happy, it has gotten him stable with parasites that he got while being fixed at five months of age. He had them for three years to no avail using the normal methods. His tummy was always hard and he was grumpy. Then he started licking my daughter after her bath because we covered her with coconut oil due to sensitive skin and it worked for her. Anyway, long story short, I had to keep shooing him away and then we would nightly just fix him his own and voilá...healed... fur is beautiful, his tummy is soft and he is a happy boy.
Holly M.

My dog Sadie had worms that I had been fighting off and on for two and a half years. I had spent lots of money on de-wormers between the vet and the pet store. That summer I was so sick of worms that I even tried horse dewormer on my poor dog, and the worms just came back within two weeks! Then my sister said that coconut oil will kill worms, so I tried it on her—the coconut oil, shredded coconut, and cloves, mixed it up with hamburger—and gave it to all my three dogs. It worked better than any dewormer I have ever used and Sadie's puppy, Poppy, who was at the time 7 or 8 months old, had the runs almost her whole life, and was constantly puking, was suddenly all better too!

Colleen

Our 6-month-old kitten was extremely lethargic and would not eat. It was the weekend and the vets were closed, and we were quite worried about him. He was a feral kitten we rescued when he was only a week old, together with his mom and littermates. He was kept in a warm safe place in our garage until being weaned and then he lived in our house and has not been outside since. Ever since he was weaned, we put a little coconut oil in his food and his coat was very soft and shiny. Now that he was sick, I decided to give him coconut oil throughout the day with a medicinal syringe. By Sunday evening he was more perky. By Monday he was even better, although he still had not eaten anything. His last meal was on Friday. Monday morning he vomited up a roundworm. We did not see any evidence of worms in his stool. On Tuesday morning he had his appetite back. We took him to the vet, but she could find nothing wrong with him. By Tuesday evening he was back to his playful self. I truly believe that it was the coconut oil that made him better.

We also give coconut oil to two of our dogs. One has colitis and it really helps to control her episodes, and the other has very bad gas problem. She still has gas, but not to the extent she had before giving her the coconut oil. I'm thinking now that we should up her dosage and see what happens.

M. G.

7

Chronic Health Problems

ALLERGIES

I knew someone who called his dog "Scratchy" because it scratched itself so often. We've all had dogs or cats that scratch themselves at times. It's only natural. However, if your pet scratches itself excessively, it may be allergic to something. Some pets are affected more at certain times of the year, while others have problems all year round. Allergies are a major cause of scratching and the number one cause of an itching rear end and subsequent scooting around on the carpet.

Our pets may be allergic to a number of things such as flea bites, pollen, mold, grasses, wool, tobacco smoke, and certain foods. Regardless of the offending agent, the main signs are scratching and chewing themselves, which may result in skin damage and secondary bacterial infections.

Allergies are triggered by an overreaction of the immune system to an otherwise harmless foreign substance referred to as an allergen. Symptoms can manifest themselves one of three ways. The most common is itching; either localized in one area or generalized (all over). Another set of symptoms may involve the respiratory tract, resulting in coughing, sneezing, wheezing, and possibly nasal or eye discharge. The third group of symptoms involves the digestive system, causing vomiting or diarrhea.

There are five known types of allergies—contact, food, bacterial, flea, and inhalant. Contact allergy is the least common of the five. It occurs when the animal comes into contact with an allergen such as a flea collar or a type of bedding. Only the area of the skin that touches the offending allergen is affected. The response is skin irritation and itching at the area of contact. Removing the irritant solves the problem, although identifying the allergen can require some detective work.

Food allergies are fairly uncommon as well. These allergies usually aren't evident in young animals but surface later, especially when the same type of food is eaten repeatedly over a long period of time. Food allergies may produce any of the clinical symptoms associated with allergies—itching, digestive disorders, and respiratory distress. The solution is to identify the offending food and remove it from the diet. Again, identifying the allergen may take some detective work. However, one clue is to look for frequently eaten foods, as they are the most likely to cause problems. Removing the suspect food should bring about relief of symptoms within a few days.

Staphylococcus (Staph) is a bacterium normally found living on dog and cat skin. We even have it on ourselves. If the animal is healthy and its skin is free of scratches, insect bites, and wounds that would provide the bacteria with an entryway inside the body, Staph poses no problems to its host. However, some pets develop an allergy to this bacterium. When this happens, the animal develops areas of inflammation and hair loss. In non-allergic animals, Staph infections are easily treated with antibiotics. However, a pet that is allergic to this bacterium will have recurrent Staph infections despite medications.

Flea allergy is very common. It is not actually the flea itself that our pets are allergic to, it's their saliva. When a flea bites a sensitive animal, its saliva triggers the allergic reaction. A normal dog or cat experiences only minor irritation in response to flea bites, often without any itching. However, a flea bite on an allergic animal can cause severe itching that can result in intense scratching and chewing and may cause the removal of a large amount of hair in the area. There will often be open sores or scabs, which can lead to secondary bacterial infections. The best solution to this problem is to keep the animal as flea-free as possible.

The most common type of allergy in dogs and cats is the inhalant type. Our pets can be allergic to all of the same inhaled allergens that affect people. These include tree, grass, and weed pollen, mold, mildew, and the house dust mite. Many of these allergies occur seasonally when plants release pollen into the air. When we breathe in these allergens, it causes respiratory problems—coughing, sneezing, runny nose, and watery eyes. We call it hay fever. Our pet's reaction, however, is usually expressed as severe generalized itching. It will chew, lick, or scratch almost any area of its body, including its feet. A common treatment is for the pet to receive allergy shots. If the allergen can be identified, very small amounts of the allergen are injected weekly. The purpose of this therapy is to reprogram the body's immune system. It is hoped that as time passes the immune system will become less reactive to the allergen.

In addition to avoiding offending allergens as much as possible, treatment for these allergies may include anti-inflammatory drugs to calm allergic reactions, shampooing and flea medication to get rid of fleas and reduce bacteria, antibiotics, and allergy shots. Interestingly, coconut oil can do all these things to help relieve allergic symptoms. Coconut oil possesses anti-inflammatory and antibacterial properties, can sooth sore, irritated skin, and can keep infection out. Coconut oil is very effective against Staph bacteria. Regular use of coconut oil can be somewhat like an allergy shot, where the animal is still exposed to allergens in the air but the effects are reduced, allowing the animal's immune system to become less reactive.

The anti-allergy effects of coconut oil led Charisa Antigua and her sister Carmina O'Conner to create CocoTherapy, a line of coconut products meant especially for pets. "We are crazy about coconut oil, and we have seen how it has helped our pets," says Charisa. "My Yorkie, Violet, was doomed to be on prednisone for life, if it were not for coconut oil. Every time I started to wean her off the prednisone, she would begin to itch and bite herself until she bled. I was heartbroken. Then one day, I put her on a regimen of coconut oil and removed all grains from her diet. Slowly she started to improve. I was able to wean her off the prednisone completely in 3 months, and she has been prednisone-free for 6 years! Her allergies are managed, and she has a long, beautiful Yorkie coat. From then on, it has been our mission to share the news and help pet owners understand the benefits of coconut oil for their pets."

Many of the success stories included in this book come from customers of CocoTherapy. These and other pet owners have found coconut oil to be an effective treatment for allergies of all kinds.

My basset hound has the worst allergies from food, seasons, and who knows what else! They cause her to get runny eyes, hot spots, dull, dry hair, and the worst is the nonstop itching. I begged my mom to just try CocoTherapy coconut oil because all other home remedies were not working. Not only does Rosie love it and talk for it during dinner time, but she has made major improvements. Her eyes don't constantly run, her hot spots haven't come back since the fall, and it has helped her itching! She loves to get oil massages and will just sleep and turn on her back so I don't miss a spot! She seems to know it helps her! If we miss a day or two you can definitely tell because her eyes get worse and the itching never stops!

Alison T.

Think Missy likes the coconut oil? She gets a belly rub, toe(s) rub every night (after she is brushed) before she goes to bed. She has stopped scratching; the allergies are controlled 99.9 percent. You can see the joy in her eyes when I set the coconut oil on the bed, she immediately jumps on the bed and says "Hurry, brush me, need my therapy!" We have a great time, she will twist and turn to get to my fingers and hands as I rub her. I let the oil melt in one hand, rub them together, she has fun going from one hand to the other.

I shudder to think of all the different medicines, the cost and the trauma I put her through this past spring and summer trying to get her some relief. I HIGHLY recommend coconut therapy for flea allergies, any allergy, scratches for our "children."

Linda B.

We have Italian Greyhounds. At one point they ranged in ages from 4 to 14 years. Two of them were brothers who were rescued. One of the brothers had lots of allergies with skin rashes that were quite itchy and bothersome. I put a little VCO in the kibble and applied it directly on his rash. I also put a little on his neck so the others would lick it off and distract him from licking the rash. The 14-year-old was preparing to leave us and though we could not keep her here for much longer, she had more energy and freedom of movement because of the soothing that VCO provided her when her digestive system was breaking down. I also use VCO and coconut water when any of them have a tummy problem. Additionally, as an artist with dogs, there are often times when a dog and paint run into one another unexpectedly. Coconut oil is very helpful in removing paint off of dog paws, ears, and even walls as it turns out.

Peggy M.

I sell your coconut oil in my store and started giving it to my dog around Christmas time. She is a 6-year-old mixed breed and has ALWAYS had terrible allergies in the spring and summer. She would rub her face on the carpet, sofa, anything available so much that she would rub the hair off around her eyes so bad she had to be put on antibiotics and Benadryl.

This is the FIRST spring that she hasn't had any sign of allergies or itching and I honestly believe it's the coconut oil. I haven't changed anything in her diet (I make her food) except the oil.

Penny Milligan

I have been using the CocoTherapy coconut oil for a few weeks now, but I can already see a difference in my dog. He has allergies and scratches a lot, and was miserable this past summer. I give him 1-2 teaspoons a day, two times a day, and he has stopped scratching and chewing his feet. I mix it with his food, although I don't have to because he would eat it right out of the jar if he could. I was skeptical at first, but now I am a believer...I also give him the coconut chips for treats, he adores it.

Gordon S.

Our Brittany spaniel had really itchy skin, around the tummy area and he used to be forever twisting round to gnaw his back near his tail. He also used to drag himself around on the concrete to scratch. We took him to the vet and they gave him a steroid injection and loaded us up with a heap of steroids, very expensive strong smelling shampoo which was meant to be left on for ten minutes (very difficult), and other meds. The vet said it was a flea allergy, although we could never find a flea on him. We didn't use any of the meds but gave the shampoo a couple of goes. No difference. Awhile later I started giving him coconut oil with his food. In about 2 weeks we noticed he'd stopped scratching and gnawing at himself. He actually stops eating when he sees me getting the coconut oil out and sits and waits for it, he loves it so much. Brilliant stuff!

Chrissy L.

85

Our kitty cat is 5 years old. We spent a THOUSAND dollars in vet bills over 4 years to treat and determine the cause of her sneezing, head congestion, sinus infections, and tests, antibiotics, and other medications. She eats 1/2-1 teaspoon of VCO every day and loves it! She stopped sneezing 50 times a day, no more discharge, no infections, and we're saving a lot of money.

Suzanne S.

I have a toy Chihuahua which suffers from allergies. I was giving her shots, and that did not work, her skin was very red and scabby...let me tell you [coconut oil] works!! I use it after bathing her, I rub it all over her body legs paws, and what a difference, no more scabs or red patches, she even smells good.

N. N.

GASTROINTESTINAL DISORDERS

Coconut oil is ideal for those who have digestive issues. It is much easier to digest than other fats and for this reason is given to hospital patients suffering from malabsorption problems who can't tolerate other fats. It is added to infant formula for the same reason. Newborn infants' digestive systems are still immature and have difficulty digesting other fats, and this is particularly true for premature infants. Coconut oil is used in hospital infant formula to help nourish them because it causes less digestive stress and is better absorbed.

The same healing effects that coconut oil demonstrates when applied topically on the skin also work inside the body, in the digestive tract. Coconut oil calms inflammation, speeds healing, fights infections, and soothes sensitive tissues. The MCFAs in coconut oil are readily absorbed into the tissues lining the digestive tract, feeding and nourishing the cells. This influx of nourishment and energy stimulates healing. As a result, some digestive problems such as constipation, diarrhea, ulcers, and colitis are greatly improved.

Our intestinal tract, as well as those of our pets, is populated by millions of bacteria and yeasts. Some of the bacteria are beneficial because they help digest our food, produce vitamins that help nourish our bodies, and in general cause us no harm. However, some of the organisms are potential troublemakers and if their populations grow too large can cause illness or digestive disorders. Large populations of the "good" bacteria crowd out the "bad" bacteria, keeping them from overpopulating the digestive tract. However, if there is an overgrowth of bad bacteria or yeasts, trouble arises, leading to various digestive complaints.

When antibiotics are taken, the drugs kill all the bacteria in the digestive system, both good and bad. This leaves a void which is quickly taken up by yeasts, such as candida. Since candida is not a bacterium, it is not affected by antibiotics. Consequently, after taking a series of antibiotics, candida populations explode, wrecking havoc on the digestive system and the body. Diet has a profound effect on the types of microorganisms populating the digestive tract. A poor diet sets in place conditions suitable for the overgrowth of bad bacteria and yeasts. Unfortunately, many pets do not have the best diets, especially if they have a low-fat diet and all they eat is dried or canned cat or dog food (see Chapter 10).

Eating coconut oil regularly can help correct and rebalance the microorganism populations of intestinal tract. The MCFAs in coconut oil kill troublesome bacteria and yeast, however, they do not harm the good bacteria. In this way, they reduce the number of bad microorganisms and allow the good bacteria to grow and take their place. The result is much better digestive function.

I have a beloved beautiful blue-eyed applehead Siamese cat who has brought so much joy to my life because of her deep affection and sweet personality towards our family. I was beside myself with grief when, at age 3, she developed a condition called megacolon where the colon can no longer push out the contents of the bowel due to loss of elasticity in the wall of the colon. Nothing can be done to reverse it and they do not know why some cats develop it. She had been fed both wet and dry foods. After a visit to the vet's office determined on x-ray she had the condition, they tried various psyllium fiber products for her to no avail, and she just continued in a downward health spiral. Next, she developed chronic cystitis due to her severely enlarge colon pressing on her bladder and could no longer urinate anything except tiny drops of blood.

Finally she was given a death sentence at the vet's and sent home to die. That week she stopped eating and eventually drinking water. I realized she was suffering from autointoxication of the bowel but

87

did not know what to do to help her. As she laid on her blanket and continued to become more and more glassy eyed, I prayed to anyone that would listen, God, Universe, etc. By this time, she had been without food for one week 2 days and water for 4 days. I tried Noni juice, as I heard it could be helpful for severe health conditions, and she just threw it back up. Now desperate, as I watched her slipping away as she had lost almost half her body weight, down to 6 pounds from her usual 11.

The next morning I woke up and she appeared to be even more depleted of life and all of a sudden coconut oil popped into my mind, miraculously. I didn't question it; I just raced to my health food store, arrived before they opened and begged them to let me in, as it was an emergency. Some emergency they must have thought, as I purchased and left with a jar of organic unrefined coconut oil.

I slightly warmed a teaspoon of the coconut oil to liquid consistency and slowly dribbled it into the side of her mouth with a little syringe I had used for other medications. I repeated this two more times; mid-afternoon and at bedtime. The next morning I was so thankful she was still alive. I repeated the [dosage of the] previous day with the coconut oil. The following morning, I was so afraid as to what I would find. When I ventured downstairs to take a peek at my little girl, she was awake, no longer almost comatose, perky even, and she wanted water and a lot of it. By afternoon she demanded food, bless her little heart.

It is now 4 years later and my precious little kitty is very healthily alive and receives her teaspoon of coconut oil every day...When I mention the coconut oil to the vets, they look at me incredulously and say 'coconut oil' with a huge question mark. Yes, coconut oil saved my kitty's life.

Lynn

I have four Yorkies and they've always had allergies and itchy skin. We've tried several medications but nothing has worked like CocoTherapy coconut oil. They are completely off medication now and their skin and coats look wonderful! One of the girls (Abby) has a sensitive tummy and always has to strain to do her business. One of the other girls (Houdina) has loose stools off and on. I read on the CocoTherapy website that the coconut chips aid in digestion *and started giving my pups the chips a couple of times each day along with coconut oil at dinner and they are doing great. They know where I keep the chips and all four of them line up for treats at least three times a day. What a difference—no more straining and no more upset tummies.*

Gina H.

One of my dogs, Caviar, has IBD (irritable bowel disease) and colitis and CocoTherapy oil and chips has really helped her. She used to vomit almost every day, and on top of that, had bloody stool with mucus. Sorry for being graphic but that's colitis for you. I thought my poor baby would have a life full of vet visits, antibiotics, flagyl, etc. On top of that she was stuck on a diet of Hills Science Diet W/D. If I took her off it, she had instant colitis. The SD W/D and flagyl helped a little with her colitis, but her IBD was getting worse. It was horrible. I cried every night. I finally went to a holistic vet, and learned about coconut oil.

I started giving her CocoTherapy coconut oil and chips with her meals. Now she is weaned off SD W/D (which is disgusting, BTW). I'm holding my breath, she has not had a bout of diarrhea or vomiting in months. No more frequent trips to the vet, or antibiotics. And no more bloody poop with slime or vomiting. I'm so thrilled. I can't stop giving it to her now, I'm scared if I stop it will come back. If I even skip giving her the coconut chips in her food for one day, her stool goes soft immediately. CocoTherapy has saved her life! My other dog Champaign also loves the coconut oil and chips. I have never seen them so healthy, happy and playful. Just amazing how these have changed their lives! I don't know how I ever managed without it. It will always be part of all my pets diet from now on.

Lisa H.

We also had a ferret that the vet wanted to put to sleep because he got sick from a blockage in his intestines, his glucose dropped and was having seizures. We did what the doctor said but added the coconut oil. Three years later he is still alive and should have died. He is blind from the seizures but happy as can be. The vet just looks at him in amazement. She said he should have died a long time ago, but we think the coconut oil saved our Ezekiel!

Jenifer U.

OVERWEIGHT

Our pets are in the midst of an epidemic. A recent headline in a major newspaper read, "Now pets have an obesity epidemic! Charity launches campaign to stop owners killing their animals with fatty foods." A 2009 national survey of veterinarians by the Association for the Prevention of Pet Obesity found that 45 percent of dogs and 58 percent of cats were overweight or obese and these numbers are rising. Pet obesity is a serious and widespread health issue. It's the most common medical condition that vets see now.

Just as in humans, extra weight in pets can lead to serious health problems, including arthritis, diabetes, kidney problems, heart problems, cancer, and a shortened lifespan. Early death is one of the consequences—two years early is the rate for dogs.

Unfortunately, many pet owners don't take this issue very seriously. Their chubby pets may even be a source of amusement. After all, a fat pet is a loved pet, right?

Molly, a 143 pound (65 kg) Rottweiler, was 50 pounds (23 kg) overweight. "I was in denial about how big Molly was," admits her owner Wayne Houlston. "We didn't realize how serious it was until she had problems with her back legs and she couldn't stand up properly." Dysplasia is a painful crippling disease characterized by deterioration of the hip joint. It is one of the most common skeletal diseases seen in dogs. Excessive body weight greatly increases the risk of developing this disease.

Jennie, a 6-year-old German shepherd-heeler mix, had always been an agile dog. But when owner, Maribeth Ashley, noticed that Jennie was having trouble getting in and out of the car for trips to the park, she was worried. Then Ashley noticed that her other dog, Pickles, also a 6-year-old shepherd mix, also needed help jumping into the car. Ashley took the dogs to her vet. The prognosis was not good. "The vet told me that they were so fat they were going to have hip dysplasia in their old age and coronary problems and all kinds of things," Ashley said.

Being overweight by only a couple of pounds may not seem all that bad, but it is much worse for our pets than it is for us. Keep in mind that just one extra pound on a six-pound toy dog is like a 125 pound person packing on 20 more pounds!

What is causing pets to become overweight? Most vets put the blame on fat. Thanks to common misperceptions about dietary fat in the human diet, most people, vets included, blame overweight problems in pets on eating too much fat. But is that really the problem? Are pet owners all of the sudden feeding their pets more fatty foods now than they did 10, 20, or 30 years ago? Not likely. People have always fed their cats and dogs table scraps; nothing new here.

However, our obsession with low-fat diets has shaped our perceptions of fat, viewing it as the cause of obesity and all of our health major health problems. This low-fat craze has carried over into the veterinary community. If pets are fat, it must be because they eat too much fat, veterinarians reason. This is their explanation for the rising epidemic in pet obesity.

Research over the past decade has shown that fat is not the culprit. The overconsumption of carbohydrates, primarily sweets and grains, is a far greater problem. Studies have clearly shown that people lose more weight on low-carb, high-fat diets than they do with high-carb, low-fat diets. Despite these studies, old ideas are hard to change and we continue to hear warnings about cutting back on our pet's fat consumption.

In an effort to curb pet obesity (and hook customers into buying new products), companies have introduced low-fat dog and cat foods. Has it done any good? No. Pet obesity continues to rise despite the availability of various low-fat products.

Although low-fat pet foods have been a commercial success, they were doomed to failure from the start in curbing the pet obesity epidemic. Commercial pet foods are already sadly deficient in fat. Lowering the fat content even more isn't going to help.

If eating excessive fat is not the cause of the obesity epidemic, what is? What has changed over the past few decades that may be the cause? Commercial pet foods have changed. Dog and cat foods used to be higher in protein and fat than they are today. Over the years, the protein and fat content has declined while the carbohydrate content has increased. When you remove fat and protein, you've got to replace it with something and that something is starchy carbohydrate—wheat, soy, potato, rice, corn, and oats. Low-fat automatically means high-carb. With this increase in carbohydrate has come an increase in obesity. Your pets won't be losing any weight on this food.

Many low-fat pet foods are 75-80 percent carbohydrate with only about 15-18 percent protein and 5-8 percent fat. These diet blends are both fat and protein deficient! This little amount of protein and fat is simply not enough for your carnivorous dog or cat. If you want to help your dog or cat lose excess weight or maintain its current proper weight, forget the low-fat diet foods and go with something that has more protein and fat. Learn to read ingredient labels and choose brands that list meat as the first ingredient. Eating junk foods and treats can also contribute to weight problems. Such foods are loaded with calories and provide little in the way of nutrition.

Of course, feeding too much of any food can encourage weight problems, so total food consumption should be monitored if weight is an issue. Nutritional researchers have known for many years that calorie restriction, to keep animals lean, improves the health of animals and increases lifespan. For example, a 2002 study published in the *Journal of the American Veterinary Medical Association* found that Labrador retrievers fed restricted-calorie diets had a median life span 2.5 years longer than non-dieting Labradors. The leaner dogs also stayed healthier in their old age.

Adding coconut oil into their diet will also help. At first this may seem surprising. The idea that fat promotes weight gain is so deeply entrenched into our minds that it is hard to believe anything different. But adding fat, particularly in the form of coconut oil, can help your pet lose excess weight.

I am frequently asked, "Won't feeding my dog coconut oil make him fat?" The answer is "No." Coconut produces energy, not body fat. As long as you are not overfeeding your pet with his other foods, you do not need to worry about giving your pet coconut oil.

Coconut oil has gained a reputation as an effective weight loss aid. One of the reasons for this is that the MCFAs in coconut oil digest differently than other fats. When you eat other fats, they go directly into circulation where they are easily deposited into fat cells and can contribute to weight gain. MCFAs, on the other hand, go directly to the liver. In the liver they are mobilized to produce energy rather than shoved into storage in fat cells. As a consequence, after eating coconut oil, you (and your pet) get a boost of energy. This energy lift actually stimulates metabolism, kicking metabolism up into a higher gear. This effect lasts for a full 24 hours. During this time the body's engines are burning at a higher rate, so more calories are being burned off. At the end of the day, fewer calories are available to be stored as fat. Therefore, if excess calories are not consumed (i.e. not overeating), you and your pet can experience weight loss. The same thing happens in our pets. Overweight pets can lose excess weight as long as they are not overfed.

What about thin pets? Will it make skinny pets skinner? No. Coconut oil has a biodirectional effect. If a pet is overweight it will help it lose excess weight. However, if it is underweight it will help improve nutrient absorption, thus promote healthy weight gain (this is due to growth of lean tissue, not *fat* buildup). It does this because coconut oil aids the body in moving in a direction towards better overall health. If that direction is to lose weight, excess fat is lost; if that direction is to gain weight, better nutrition accomplishes that.

Love, love LOVE coconut oil for my dogs! Both are rescue dogs, one was VERY overweight (they only fed her junk food and didn't allow her outdoors for 3 years because they weren't allowed to have a dog where they lived). The coconut oil helped her weight regulate when NOTHING else would! No more bad breath in either dog, all skin issues cleared up (even scarring from cigarette burns is fading!). Both dogs smell neutral even after running outdoors! Coats are soft and shiny, the list goes on! Small dogs, so we worked up to 1 teaspoon per day, per dog. Wonderful!
Anonymous

Helps to trim down a thick canine waistline. Coconut oil is gaining respect for being a fat burning food. I've been feeding my Shelties about a tablespoon on their food and they have lost that roll of belly fat.
N. N.

This is what my dogs are eating tonight. Raw meat, cooked pumpkin and fresh coconut cream. They only get the cream if I am using it for cooking or making oil. Otherwise I just sprinkle some oil onto their food. I changed their diet a few months ago when the older dog became quite ill. She was obese after years of eating kibble. On this diet she has lost 3 kg (7 lb) which is a lot for a dog who weighed 9 kg (20 lb) and she has changed from a cranky old dog to being happy and playful again. She also has a long history of skin

problems which disappeared almost immediately with application of coconut oil.
Annabella D.

I do know that coconut oil has done wonders for my golden retriever who has lots of allergies. His entire stomach area cleared up, he has lot more energy, and he has lost weight!"
Maureen W.

BONES AND JOINTS
When added to foods, coconut oil improves the assimilation of vitamins and minerals that are present in the foods. Minerals such as calcium and magnesium, which are essential for good bone and joint health, are better absorbed from foods when coconut oil is eaten at the same time.

The type of fat in pet foods plays a significant role in bone and joint health. Researchers at Purdue University found that free radicals generated from oxidized (rancid) vegetable oils interfere with bone formation, contributing to osteoporosis. They discovered that antioxidants such as vitamin E can inhibit the destructive action of free radicals. Coconut oil, being a highly saturated fat, is extremely resistant to oxidation, so much so that it functions much like a protective antioxidant. The combination of improved mineral absorption and protection against bone damaging free radicals supports the growth of strong bones and healthy joints.

Adding coconut oil into your pet's diet can make dramatic improvements in bone and joint health. Beverly's nine-year-old Shar Pei dog, Taz, suffered from severe arthritis in its hips and "almost non-existent front elbows." She asked her veterinarian if there was any treatment that might help. "No, the dog's condition was irreversible," she was told. Nothing could help. Recovery was "impossible." The veterinarian suggested they put the dog down because he needed both front and rear legs to stay mobile. It wouldn't be long before the dog was totally immobile. Although heartbroken, Beverly wasn't a person who takes "impossible" for an answer and began researching for a solution. She learned about coconut oil and decided to give it a try. After only two weeks of taking 1 tablespoon of coconut oil daily, "Taz was up and running like a puppy on all four legs," says Beverly. "It has been over a year, and he's still truckin'."

I have a 12-year-old all white cat named Zoe. She is getting arthritis in her back hips and does very little jumping anymore and she limped when she walked. Every morning she likes to get a drink out of the bathroom faucet while I am getting ready for my day. My ritual is putting coconut oil all over my skin. Zoe is my audience during this ritual. So I put a little chunk on my finger and I was surprised how much she liked it. I am talking about a piece about the size of a pencil eraser. Then after eating it she would run off. This became her ritual every morning with me. She has more energy and she stopped limping. She makes smaller jumps with ease. I believe she knows this helps her, she is a smart cat.

Deby L.

My large bulldog had severe hip problems. I gave him two glucosamine and one coconut oil capsule every day. He is so much better. I took him walking today for the first time in a long time. We have always had him on glucosamine but we have never had this kind of result.

Deborah

Casey is a Chihuahua mix given to me as a gift when she was young. Her hind knees are a bit knobby and the vet said we would have to watch them as she has a loose ligament in them and she may eventually need surgery. She was hesitant to jump up on the couch or bed and we often assisted her by picking her up. Even though she was a young dog she acted much older. I began putting virgin coconut oil on her food and it was no time that she began springing up onto everything! The vet was amazed.

S. F.

CANCER

Coconut oil has potent anti-cancer properties. In studies evaluating the effect that various dietary oils have on tumor growth and development in animals, coconut oil was found to significantly stunt tumor growth in comparison to other oils. For example, in one study the effect of dietary oils on mammary (breast) cancer was examined. Researchers used a variety of different oils—olive oil, corn oil, canola oil, safflower oil, and coconut oil. The animals were fed an identical diet, except for the type of oil. Each animal was exposed to powerful carcinogenic chemicals to induce mammary cancer. All of the animals developed tumors, except those given coconut oil. Tissue samples were taken and examined, but the investigators could find no trace of cancer.

Interestingly, the animals that developed the largest and most numerous tumors were the ones fed polyunsaturated vegetable oils. Other researchers who performed similar studies with various oils had the similar results. Coconut oil or MCFAs seem to block tumor growth, while polyunsaturated vegetables oils (corn, soybean, safflower, etc.) encouraged it.

Other researchers have found that coconut oil strengthens immune function. It does this in part by increasing white blood cell production in the bone marrow. White blood cells are the workhorse of our immune system. Coconut oil can also improve red blood cell production, which can help treat anemia. For these reasons, coconut oil and MCFAs have been recommended for cancer patients undergoing chemo and radiation therapies, which destroy bone marrow and lead to anemia and low immune function. With the addition of coconut oil in the diet, many of the adverse side effects associated with cancer therapy can be reduced or eliminated.

Whether as an accompaniment to conventional or natural cancer therapies or as part of a cancer prevention plan, coconut oil can provide significant protection.

My dogs and I have taken and tried tons of supplements, I can't even keep track of how many we've tried in the past. I'm a health nut and have been experimenting with natural and holistic health supplements for over 23 years. Out of all the supplements I've tried, I've never tried one like CocoTherapy coconut oil. I was doubtful at first, a lot of the health claims seemed too good to be true, but now I've been converted! It has proven itself so many times for so many ailments, when nothing else worked. I not only use it for my pets, I use it for myself, for virtually everything.

My dogs and I have never felt and looked better since we all started taking coco oil! It's delicious as well, we both love the taste! I now recommend it to all my health nut friends! My sister's Golden mix, Shelby, was diagnosed with canine lymphoma. She underwent chemotherapy, which resulted in a lowering in her white blood cells. Her vet recommended a special diet, which included coconut oil. Coconut oil helps to support the immune system, support her digestive system, gives her necessary energy, and at the same time has a negative effect on tumor growth.

Shelby had been lethargic, lost her appetite, and seemed very depressed. She was also nauseated, and had diarrhea. When my sister added CocoTherapy coconut oil to her diet, Shelby's appetite increased, she seemed to gain her strength, her nausea and vomiting subsided, and her playfulness returned. She now goes on her daily walks and is interested in treats again. She loves CocoTherapy coconut chips too. There are studies too that show that coconut oil can prevent renegade cells from going "cancerous." Shelby is now in remission, and with the addition of coconut oil in her diet, hopefully will remain in remission and will help to prevent other cancer cells from forming.

Dan O.

I have a 10-year-old basset hound that was bit by a rattlesnake 2 years ago. He smells horribly from the bacteria inside him from the snake's fangs. He is also starting to grow tumors that basset hounds typically get with age. I started giving him some coconut oil on his food about 4 months ago. The rumors have started to shrink, he has more energy, and the smell is slowly going away.

Jenifer U.

My collie had a month to live. Cancer in his mouth. I started rubbing coconut oil into his gums all day, every day. It cleared up all the sores except for one. A year later he is still kicking and feels fine.

Wendy V.

The veterinarian said it looked like a tumor and he recommended immediate surgery. I figured that if coconut oil is good for humans, it should be good for animals as well, so I began applying it to the lump on my dog's forehead. As time passed, the lump grew smaller and smaller and eventually disappeared. It never returned. We avoided the surgery.

L. J.

DEGENERATIVE DISEASES

Coconut oil has a remarkable rejuvenating effect on our pets. Even very serious health problems may improve with the use of coconut oil, as the following stories show.

Diabetes

I know many people with both type I and type II diabetes who have been helped by using coconut oil. They started slowly and increased the amount used with meals slowly while monitoring their sugar. I personally had the wonderful experience of helping a friend who had a very sick diabetic dog get off of insulin. We added coconut oil to her daily routine. With our treatment we lowered her insulin demand by 85 percent in 3-4 days, and off from it entirely in about 2 weeks. It really was a miracle.

I use it every day for Shamus, it brought his sugar levels down. Been using it for 2 years. It is available in Walmart, GNC, and I am sure other stores.

K. M.

I bought the refined coconut oil for my three large dogs. I had read that the refined coconut oil has much the same properties/values as the virgin coconut oil (VCO), though it has no taste. My dogs are older dogs: one, my black lab, has diabetes and cataracts. I give him insulin shots 2 times daily and drops to dissolve his cataracts. He was having trouble getting up and trembled when he walked. Since the coconut oil treatment—2 tablespoons daily on his food, he no longer trembles, walks more than he could before and has lost weight.

T. S.

Cataracts

My friend has a shin tzu dog which had cataracts in its eyes. Actually the dog came from his sister-in-law who could not take care of the dog properly with its vision limitation. My friend put virgin

98

coconut oil on both eyes twice a day. After about a month its sight was restored.

Tony

Pancreatic Disorder

My dog was diagnosed with possible exocrine pancreatic insufficiency. While researching this condition I came across coconut oil. I got extremely interested in it and purchased some of the oil along with three of Dr. Fife's books. Bertie, my dog, loves the coconut oil. Because of the illness he only weighed 40 pounds and needed to put on a lot more weight. For 10 days I have been giving him the equivalent of about 2 tablespoons a day throughout the day and his weight has improved and so has his digestion. When I took him back to the vets for a follow-up exam he was clear! He has been very close to it on his first test. I am convinced the coconut oil played a very large role in his recovery. He is now as healthy as can be.

V. S.

Hypothyroidism

If your dog is taking thyroid medication, you may need to gradually lower it and eventually discontinue using it when coconut oil is given regularly.

I have three dogs, all 100+ pounds, and they get 1½ tbsp in the am, and another 1½ tbsp in the evening. They love it and it has worked wonders for them. My malamute, who has a thyroid problem, recently went from being hypothyroid to being hyperthyroid (which has never happened since he was diagnosed 5 years ago), and I have lowered his thyroid medication to just once a day.

Val

Our dog Maggie was diagnosed with "borderline hypo-thyroidism," by two separate vets, on two separate occasions. "Borderline hypothyroidism," also called "subclinical" or "low-normal" hypothyroidism, is a condition where the dog is definitely suffering from a weakened thyroid system, but it is not yet severe enough to register out of the "normal range." In borderline cases, the conventional treatment is to provide the pet with a small thyroid supplement for 30 days just to see if it improves. However, there are risks in this approach. If thyroxine levels become too high, other body organs can be damaged. As we were not prepared to take this risk, and with the advice of a holistic vet, we added coconut oil to Maggie's diet, as coconut oil is known to help support healthy thyroid function. We then had Dr. Jean Dodds, the foremost authority on canine hypothyroidism at "Hemopet," run her thyroid tests. We are happy to report, that Maggie's result showed that she no longer had borderline hypothyroidism.

Anonymous

Mystery Illness

In some cases, coconut oil has the ability to restore health even when an animal appears to be at death's doorstep.

About a week after we moved into our new home, our eight-year-old dog, Davis got deathly ill. We actually thought he may have broken his back on the stairs. He would not walk and had to be carried everywhere. The vet was certain that he had hurt his back as well, but on the second day, he started having blisters on his feet and on the back of his body. When he stood up on his feet, they would just bleed. (Just lovely in the new house!) After inconclusive tests, as well as even a spinal tap, they decided to call it an immune disease. Still not sure quite the diagnosis, but he was on death's bed. After $1500 in tests and medications the vet still was unsure of prognosis and suggested to put him out of his misery. Davis was still unable to walk, but now unable to open one eye and had large half-dollar size lesions all over his back and hind legs.

After making the appointment on Friday to put him to sleep on Monday, I decided to try one last thing over the weekend. I read on the net about coconut oil being good for dog's immune system. Desperately I tried it, and miraculously about four hours after his first dose, he got up and walked. Within a day, his feet stopped bleeding and he was once again walking over to the food bowel! I am convinced—and just amazed! Funny how after $1500 of tests and meds from the vet, a $15 jar of coconut oil healed him! It has now been two weeks and he is back to normal.

L. H.

8

Dementia and Age Related Conditions

COGNITIVE DYSFUNCTION SYNDROME

Most pets age much faster than we do. Dogs and cats age about seven times faster; one year to us is equivalent to about seven years to them. This rule of thumb is just an approximation. Dogs and cats mature quicker early in their lives and then aging slows down after they reach adulthood. A dog or cat is essentially a full adult after about 1½ years. At two years of age a small dog or cat is the equivalent of a human at about 24 years of age. At ten years, they are in their mid 50s, at 15 years, mid 70s, and at 20 years, mid 90s. Larger dogs age faster than smaller dogs, so they would be in their 90s several years sooner. Small dogs can live upward to 20 years. Medium and large dogs generally live 12 to 13 years.

As our pets age, like us they become less active, tire quicker, sleep more, are not as strong, and lack the endurance they had in their youth. These are all normal conditions of aging and should be expected. Unfortunately, with age, many of our pets develop age-related health problems such as diabetes, cataracts, arthritis, and such. Of these, probably none are as heartbreaking as dementia. It is sad to see a once active, loving dog digress, losing all sense of awareness and even its personality. He no longer rushes excitedly to greet you when you come into the room, stops responding to his name, or may even growl at you or other family members as if meeting a stranger. It's painful to pet owners to witness the mental decline.

My 14+ year old rescue dachshund has had dementia for a year. She's lost interest in almost everything she used to enjoy. She paces and is lost when she's awake so she's confined to two rooms unless we are with her. She sleeps almost all day but is up in the night, pacing and panting. That is the hardest to deal with. Several prescribed meds have been tried to help with the sleeping with limited success, have had about the same luck with OTC meds. I'm hand feeding her a good quality food. She's arthritic and has a great deal of difficulty walking. She has a med for that. She doesn't respond to her name. We question her vision, although the vet said she can see, at least large objects. I'm always alert to when she's been out, to try to prevent accidents. The time is near when I'll have to let her go. It will break my heart. The grand kids love her so much.

Mary B.

Molly is my 15-year-old border collie, she's in pretty good health however over the last few months I have seen a dramatic change in her behavior, constantly wants out but when she gets out just stands there not knowing. She's asking for food all the time, I think she forgets that she has been well fed. If I leave the room she freaks out and will pace the house looking for me. She stares into space and now goes to the wrong side of the door when trying to get out. I know I'm going to have to make the hardest decision of my life, I wish nature would make the decision from me.

G. S.

Today my 8-year-old Jack Russell was diagnosed with dementia, I'd never heard of it in dogs and was in utter shock, but it explained so many of her odd behaviors. She no longer wants anyone to touch her, she is also nervous of doors, urinating indoors and I thought that I had done something wrong. It's breaking my heart, she was always an affectionate dog and so loved by us all. It's not her time yet but I am dreading that moment. I just wanna cuddle her and keep her safe but I know there is nothing I can do for her to make it better. It is tormenting me.

Nikki

Each of these dogs is suffering from cognitive dysfunction syndrome (CDS). This condition, once called senile or old dog syndrome, causes mental changes that are very similar to Alzheimer's disease in humans. Autopsies of affected dogs reveal the same type of degenerative brain lesions seen in Alzheimer's patients.

Disorientation and confusion are some of the principal symptoms. The dog may wander about the house or yard as if lost, get stuck in corners or under or behind furniture, have difficulty finding the door or stand at the hinge side or go to the wrong door, not recognize familiar people, and fail to respond to verbal cues or its own name. Activity and sleep patterns are disturbed. The dog sleeps more, especially during the day, but less at night. There is a decrease in purposeful activity and an increase in aimless wandering and pacing. Dogs may also exhibit compulsive behavior with circling, tremors, stiffness, and weakness. Interactions with family members decline. The dog shows less enthusiasm upon greeting family members, doesn't wag its tail like it used to, and may walk away when being petted. House training skills become lost. The dog may urinate and defecate indoors, sometimes even in the view of owners, and may forget to signal to go outside.

A study by the Animal Behavior Clinic at the University of California, Davis revealed that 28 percent of dogs aged 11 to 12 years and 68 percent of dogs aged 15 to 16 years showed one or more signs of CDS. Although most studies of CDS have focused on the condition in dogs, cats are affected as well. However, the percentage of affected cats is much lower.

Ever since I found her lying in a pile of snow 16 years ago my 19-year-old cat, Lucy has been my best friend. No matter what I've been through in life I could always count on coming home to her waiting at the door for me. She doesn't do that anymore. She now spends her time either sleeping or wandering the apartment making very loud, continuous meowing noises. She stares at 'nothin' and doesn't even notice me when I walk up to her until I touch her, then she sort of jumps as if startled. Sometimes she can hear me, other times she can't. I had my sister's dog over here last night and Lucy,

Warning Signs of Canine Dementia

Disorientation and confusion: Appears lost or confused in the house or yard. Fails to recognize familiar people. Fails to respond to verbal cues or name. Has difficulty finding the door or stands on the hinge side of the door or stands at wrong door to go outside. Appears to forget the reason for going outdoors. Gets stuck in corners, or under or behind furniture.

Decreased Interaction with family members: Seeks attention less often. Walks away when being petted. Shows less enthusiasm upon greeting you. No longer greets family members.

Sleep and activity changes: Sleeps more during the day and more overall in a 24-hour period. Sleepless during the night. Shows increase in aimless activity by wandering or pacing more.

Loss of house-training: Urinates or defecates indoors. Has accidents indoors soon after being outside. Forgets to ask to go outside.

who normally would swat at other animals, walked right up to the dog as if she didn't even recognize what it was. She eats and drinks much more than normal but before she'll even take a drink of water she will put her head in the glass and meow to it for a long time as if she's singing it a song. I don't know what to do. I love that cat.

Sean

I've had Lucy since I was 8 and she has always been so easy to take care of. The only medical issue we ever had was seasonal allergies that required eye drops. Now, however, she seems to have trouble jumping and running and at night I've always let her in my room no problem but she's begun crying 4-5 hours after I fall asleep. This isn't her normal meow but sounds more like she's mewling "hello." It's awful sounding but I think she just gets lonely or scared. Finally, after being checked for infection and all, I've learned she's lost some of her litter box training. I've added a second box to her room and am obsessive about cleaning which has helped, but at

Warning Signs of Feline Dementia

Disorientation and confusion: Gets trapped in corners or behind furniture. Has difficulty locating the litter box.

Forgetting the location of the litter box: Forgets years litter box training with inappropriate urination or defecation.

Change in sleeping patterns: Days and nights become mixed, sleeping all day and active at night.

Decreased grooming: Lack of interest in keeping coat in good condition.

Behavioral changes: Increased irritability or anxiety. More aggressive or seeks more attention. May not appear to recognize family members. Loss of interest in playful activities. Aimless wandering or pacing or reduced activity.

Decreased appetite: Forgets to eat or lacks usual interest in food. Usually eats less, but may eat more because they have forgotten they have already eaten.

Loud vocalizations: Increased or excessive loud vocalizations, especially at night.

what point do I put her down? I'm still joking with friends that she can vote! I hope she goes easy and naturally in her sleep.
   Lisa

   The symptoms of CDS in cats are in many ways similar to those in dogs. The most pronounced symptom is confusion and disorientation. Cats will often stare blindly into space or at a wall. They may not recognize family members or other pets, and they may become stressed under ordinary conditions. They begin to sleep more than usual, especially during the day, but may be up at night wandering about, often meowing. One of the most characteristic symptoms is loud or odd vocalizations. All cats have a certain level of "talkativeness." Some are fairly quiet while others meow about everything. With CDS there is an increase in vocalizations that can become excessive. This behavior is more common at night, which may wake up the household. Loss of grooming habits and litter box training is typical. Some cats, by their nature, can be a little cantankerous, but when affected by CDS their behavior may change and they may become increasingly irritable or easily provoked. Appetite may decrease and they may even forget to eat.

A study by G.M. Landsberg and colleagues at the North Toronto Animal Clinic in Canada indicated that 28 percent of pet cats aged 11 to 14 years developed at least one sign consistent with CDS, and this increased to over 50 percent for cats 15 years of age or older.

There are few treatment options for CDS. The most commonly used drug is Anipryl (selegiline, L-deprenyl), which is also used to treat Parkinson's disease in humans and has been found to improve some symptoms associated with CDS. Anipryl is currently the only FDA-approved drug for the treatment of CDS in dogs. There is no drug approved for the treatment of CDS in cats.

Anipryl works by stimulating the production of dopamine—a chemical that transmits nerve impulses in the brain. The drug is given once daily as a pill. While this drug may improve some symptoms, it doesn't work for all dogs and carries risk of adverse side effects. Side effects reported include vomiting, diarrhea, hyperactivity/restlessness, anorexia, muscle weakness, diminished hearing, heart and lung problems, loss of coordination, staggering, disorientation, and seizures, among others. Some of these symptoms are similar to those caused by the disease itself! Even in those dogs that do show improvement, anipryl does not stop the progression of the disease because it does not address the underlying problem. There's got to be a better solution. And there is.

SUPERFUEL FOR THE BRAIN

For years veterinarians attributed the symptoms of senility to be a normal part of aging. However, many pets live well into old age without experiencing any appreciable loss in mental function. Continued scientific advances have shown that while age is a risk factor, it is not the cause. Alzheimer's, as well as CDS, are diseases and are not a normal part of aging. The brains of dogs that age normally are much different from the brains of those affected by CDS. While there may be many factors that contribute to CDS, the underlying cause is a defect in glucose metabolism.

The energy that powers the mind and the body comes from the carbohydrate, fat, and protein in the foods consumed. The primary source of fuel for the cells is glucose, which comes primarily from the carbohydrate in plant foods like grains and vegetables. Meat, too, can supply glucose. About 50 percent of the protein consumed can be converted into glucose. The rest is used to build and maintain muscle and other tissues. Dietary fat cannot be converted into glucose to any appreciable degree but is broken down into fatty acids which, like glucose, can be burned as fuel. The cells use either glucose or fatty acids to supply their energy needs.

Recent human and animal research has shown that Alzheimer's is caused by the inability of the neurons or brain cells to effectively convert glucose into energy. Without energy, the neurons die, the brain shrinks, and memory and cognitive function decline. As the brain loses its ability to metabolize glucose, it slowly degenerates into dementia.

In the wild, animals, and especially carnivores such as dogs and cats may go for days without eating. In such cases blood glucose levels drop dramatically. Fatty acids from stored fat then supply most of the energy needed by the cells in the body, with one exception—the brain. Fatty acids for the most part are blocked from entering the brain by the blood-brain barrier. The brain is the most important organ in the body, so its health and survival is of extreme importance. To preserve brain health when food consumption is low, an alternative fuel source is used. When blood glucose levels drop, the liver begins to convert stored fat into a special type of fuel called *ketone bodies* or *ketones*. They are referred to as "superfuel" for the brain because they produce more energy than either glucose or fatty acids. It is like putting high octane fuel into the gas tank of your car—you get more horsepower and better gas mileage.

Unlike fatty acids, ketones can easily pass through the blood-brain barrier and feed the brain. During times of low food consumption, ketones supply most of the energy needs of the brain. Almost every cell in the body can use ketones for energy, but they are absolutely essential for the brain. Ordinarily, blood ketone levels are very low. The liver only produces them when glucose levels drop too low to adequately power the brain.

In addition to being a superior energy source, ketones also trigger the activity of certain survival-promoting proteins in the brain called *brain derived neurotrophic factors*. These proteins regulate growth, function, and the ability of neurons to make neurotransmitters—the chemical signals that allow brain cells to communicate with each other and to store and retrieve memories. They also play a significant role in the maintenance, repair, and growth of brain cells.

Ketones provide the key to overcoming CDS. Ketones bypass the defect in glucose metabolism in the brain seen in CDS, providing the neurons with the energy they need to function properly and stimulate repair and healing.

Ordinarily, ketone production is triggered by low blood glucose levels. This happens only when food, and especially carbohydrate, consumption is extremely low. This can happen with complete food restriction (starvation), which of course is impractical, or it can happen with a controlled diet consisting of only meat and fat, particularly fatty organ meats. Fat is very important because it does not supply any of the glucose that would turn off the ketone production process, plus it supplies the fatty acids needed to synthesize ketones. Meat consumption would need to be limited because too much meat can also raise glucose levels. Most commercial dog foods are composed primarily of high-carb ingredients such as corn, soy, or wheat and would need to be completely eliminated. A diet rich in fatty organ and muscle meats and low in carbohydrate is a natural diet for dogs. It's no wonder it would also be therapeutic and prolong brain health.

COCONUT KETONES

Another approach is also possible. In recent years, a certain group of dietary fats have been identified that are converted into ketones regardless of blood glucose levels. These fats are known as medium chain triglycerides (MCTs). When consumed, they go directly to the liver. In the liver, some are burned immediately to produce energy while others are converted into ketones. This conversion is independent of blood glucose levels or any other nutrients present in the diet. Adding MCTs to your pet's diet can raise blood ketone levels to therapeutic levels and basically accomplish the same thing as a strict meat and fat diet.

In 2008 researchers from the University of Toronto seeking new treatments for Alzheimer's found that adding MCTs into the diet could help prevent and even stop the degenerative processes that lead to CDS in dogs and Alzheimer's in humans. They found that aged dogs that were given a diet that included MCTs had much healthier brains. The researchers stated the brains showed "dramatically improved" energy metabolism and experienced much less damage compared to aged dogs that were not given the MCTs.[1]

Another group of researchers found that adding MCTs to dog chow resulted in improved daytime activity, increased performance on visual-spatial memory tasks and motor learning tasks, increased short-term memory, and increased probability of learning tasks.[2] What was interesting about this study was that it showed that MCTs not only slow down memory loss but can also bring about improvement. This suggests that MCTs not only prevent and stop brain degeneration, but can even reverse it! So there is hope for those animals that have already developed CDS.

All dogs and cats can benefit from the addition of MCTs in their diet regardless of their age. In 2010 the *British Journal of Nutrition* published a study sponsored by pet food maker Purina and conducted by researchers from the University of Toronto. At the beginning of the study, aged Beagle dogs were subjected to a battery of cognitive tests, which were used to establish a baseline of cognitive ability. The dogs in the treatment group were then placed on a diet supplemented with 5.5 percent MCTs for eight months, during which all the dogs were tested with a series of cognitive tests to assess learning ability, egocentric visuospatial function (thought processes that involve visual and spatial awareness) and attention. The MCT-supplemented group showed significantly better performance in most of the test protocols in comparison to the control group. This study demonstrated that long-term supplementation with MCTs is safe and can have a very positive effect on cognitive ability. You can start animals on coconut oil early in life so that they can avoid or reduce the risk of dementia-related problems in the future.

Dementia does not happen overnight. It's a long process that takes years before it becomes evident. Small changes that affect behavior and cognitive ability occur over time, such as becoming slower and less alert. This can easily be attributed to normal aging.

"Cognitive decline is usually a slow and gradual process with owners not noticing any significant changes until their dog is about 12 years old," said Dr. Jill Cline, senior research nutritionist at Purina. "But by the time your dog has changed in behavior it may be hard to do anything about it. Prevention is always better than cure so therefore it's best to start feeding a senior diet with anti-aging [MCTs] from about seven years of age." Better yet would be to include coconut oil in your pet's food as early as possible to prevent problems later on.[3]

A simple step pet owners can take to prevent and treat CDS is to add a source of MCTs to their dog's or cat's food. By far, the richest natural source of MCTs is found in coconut oil. Coconut oil consists of 63 percent MCTs. A spoonful a day is all that is needed to produce therapeutic levels of ketones. For treatment purposes for pets that are showing signs of dementia, use 1-2 teaspoons (5-10 g) of coconut oil for every 5 pounds (2.5 kg) of body weight. If your dog weighs 20 pounds (9 kg), give it 4-8 teaspoons (20-40 g) of coconut oil. For best results, divide this amount into two equal doses and give one in the morning and the other in the late afternoon or early evening. In this case, each dose would equal 2 teaspoons (10 g). The oil can be mixed into the dog chow or given as is. Most dogs and cats love the taste of coconut oil and will readily lick it off a spoon. Be aware that these dosages are for the treatment of dementia and are different from the maintenance and treatment dosages given in the following chapter.

Combining coconut oil with a healthy low-carb diet will improve the effectiveness of the treatment. High-fat, low-carb diets are natural for cats and dogs. In fact, the primary cause of CDS in carnivorous animals, like dogs and cats, is consuming too much carbohydrate such as grains and soy and too little good quality fat. See Chapters 10 and 11 for more information about natural healthy diets. Changing the diet can have a dramatic effect.

My Molly (Norwegian Forest Cat) is almost 16 now. Recently I have noticed her staring off into space, she is becoming antisocial and pooping on the floor on occasions, sleeping about 23 hours a day. Since I do not take medications and refuse to put chemicals in my body, I did not think she should have chemicals either. So I

decided to take her to a holistic vet. With her help we did a total detox and cleanse and put her on an organic raw diet and herbal supplements. The change has been profound, she sleeps less and is much happier and actually playing, which she had not done in years. Right now I am hopeful to have a few more good years with Molly. I would recommend to everyone dealing with a pet with dementia to have your pet evaluated and seek advice from a holistic vet.
    JG

Drugs are not the answer. They cannot cure CDS or any disease for that matter. However, a good diet along with coconut oil can work wonders. This approach is not only effective for CDS but also for other neurological disorders such as epilepsy, degenerative myeopathy (deterioration of nerves in the spinal cord), head trauma, and others—all of which can affect dogs and cats. Dietary changes and coconut oil have proven to be successful in reversing a variety of neurological disorders in humans. If you would like more information on how coconut oil can successfully treat similar conditions in humans, I recommend reading my book *Stop Alzheimer's Now.*

AGE RELATED CONDITIONS

Not only can coconut oil help with dementia, but it can also improve such age-related conditions as low energy, dry skin, dull coat, loss of mobility, lack of interest and enthusiasm, less attention to grooming, and frequent accidents indoors.

Coconut oil can boost your pet's energy levels, improve its health, and restore much of your pet's youthful love for life. The ketones produced from coconut oil are a super potent source of fuel that can be used by most cells and organs in the body. Ketones increase oxygen utilization while increasing energy output, thus enhancing the cell's efficiency. For example, in comparison to glucose, ketones increase the hydraulic output of the heart by an incredible 28 percent! With a better source of fuel, the heart functions better, as well as the brain and other muscles and organs. This can have a dramatic revitalizing effect on an aged animal. Coconut oil can add not just years to your dog's or cat's life but functional, happy years.

I have a 17 month old Pomeranian who gets dry skin and ear infections...Coconut oil has done nothing but WONDERS for both of my dogs. In fact, my other dog, who is mixed, had three strokes, wobbling, arthritis, vestibular, etc., and the vet wanted to put him to sleep, but I refused! I have given him virgin coconut oil for six months and he has improved dramatically 95 percent there, and the vet is surprised. BTW, he's 18 years. My Pomeranian's skin is no longer dry and his coat is luxurious...I make coconut icicles for them to eat and enjoy. They adore it. No vet, no vet bills to pay, dogs are happy and healthier – and I'm extremely happy with it. I take it myself, too.

Lynn

My dogs are older; one, my black lab, has diabetes and cataracts. I give him insulin shots two times daily and drops to dissolve his cataracts. He was having trouble getting up and trembled when he walked. Since the coconut oil treatment—2 tablespoons daily on his food—he no longer trembles, walks more than he could before and has lost weight. I have cut back on his food as he doesn't seem to want his past amount.

T. J.

My neighbor has a female Doberman that they adore. She became very ill and could not stand. Their vet said Dobermans often develop "wobblers" and there was not much they could do. It was degenerative and she may have about a month to live. They were, of course, crushed. I, of course, never gave up and told him to add virgin coconut oil to her food. I sent my neighbor home with a small jar of the precious oil. He was willing to try anything. They were having to force feed her a liquid diet at the time. In 24 hours the dog was up! Over the course of the week she continued to improve. He now puts it in her food daily. She no longer wobbles when she walks and all is right with the world! My neighbor was amazed.

S. F.

About 3 weeks ago someone asked if it was OK to feed coconut milk to dogs, I Googled and found a wealth of information on the health benefits of coconut flesh, milk, and especially coconut oil for both humans and dogs. Some of the claims were that the oil was anti-fungal, anti-bacterial, that it contained a particularly good form of fat, that it increases the metabolism, that this in turn helps with thyroid issues and diabetes and possibly aids those with Alzheimer's.

Since it is a safe food source and can be used as a cooking oil or eaten uncooked, I decided to experiment...on Barney. Barney has arthritis, two fatty lumps, one of which affects his gait but which the vet does not wish to remove because of his age and its position. He has lost a lot of his zest, is stiff and sedentary and consequently puts on weight which is hard to shift. He has also begun to develop odd superstitions and worries about floor surfaces, bridges and walking on shiny things.

Day one, I started with a very small amount as the advice for dogs was that too much too soon would cause greasy stools and be unhelpful. Day one Barney cantered past Beth causing her jaw to drop open. It wasn't a sustained run but it was more powerful than anything he had done for months.

Day two he was back to annoying me at tea-time, bringing me toys and poking me with them. Again this was behaviour that had become increasingly rare. By the end of the first week Barney was moving more freely some of the time, he was not pestering me for food at odd times of the day. He was leaving some of his meals, but had more energy for general pottering about during the day.

By the second week, his coat was looking and feeling more lustrous, the slight whiff of old dog and things he might have sat in was going, and the small bump on his head, a spot the vet asked us to keep our eyes on, had disappeared.

By the third week he was jumping well into the car and out again. He was still not a young dog but he was able to enjoy his walks and alternate his speed and initiate play with Beth now and then. He reverted to his old behaviour of finding plastic bottles in the park and shoving them up my bottom, who ever thought that would please me! The whites of his eye are brighter, his stance is more upright and best of all other people have commented on how changed he seems. I did think perhaps it was the weather then the change in the weather then anything but the oil but I am now pretty sure that it is doing him some good and making his senior years more enjoyable for him and for me.

Celia

After reading this far into this book, you may be getting the impression that coconut oil is a wonder food that can cure all ills. I would like to clearly state that coconut oil is not a cure-all. It can help with many health problems to a degree that in many ways is superior to commercial products and drugs designed to treat these problems, but it cannot cure all problems. Its effectiveness can also vary depending on your pet's diet. Combined with a good diet, coconut oil can seemingly work miracles. If the diet is poor, however, there is only so much coconut oil can do. For example, if your pet is suffering from a mineral deficiency, coconut oil might help with some of the symptoms, but it cannot address the underlying problem—lack of minerals. Only getting the missing minerals can cure this problem. There are dozens of vitamins and minerals necessary for obtaining and maintaining good health; some say as many as 60 major and trace minerals are required for optimal health. Coconut oil alone has limited effect when the diet is severely deficient.

The question we now ask is: what constitutes a good diet? Is kibble considered a good diet? It has been formulated by scientists to meet nutritional requirements, hasn't it? What about more costly foods like the Science Diet or a raw food diet? Or how about human foods and table scraps? These questions are answered in the following chapters.

9

How to Use
Coconut Oil

Coconut oil and other coconut products are rapidly growing in popularity among people and their pets. Even pet food manufacturers are recognizing the value of coconut and are starting to put it into their products. Some brands already on the market include PowerStance, Nature's Variety, and Purina Pro Plan Senior 7+ Original. CocoTherapy sells pure coconut oil and coconut chips marketed specifically for pets; their products are "food grade" so that pet owners can enjoy these products themselves.

Coconut oil is available at all health food stores, including vitamin shops like GNC and Vitacost, and on the Internet. Some pet stores carry it (look for CocoTherapy). Some major grocery chains are also beginning to stock it, such as Walmart, Kroger, and Costco.

Fresh mature coconuts and canned coconut milk are sold in most all grocery stores. Look in the produce section for fresh coconuts and the ethnic section for coconut milk. Do not buy the coconut milk "beverages" sold in the refrigerated section of the store. These are not pure coconut milk but have water, sugar, and flavorings added. They are meant only for humans. Grocery stores also sell desiccated or dried coconut, but the type they sell almost always has added sugar and preservatives. You can get unsweetened, chemical-free dried coconut at your local health food store.

Coconut water, which some people like to give to their pets for its rehydration properties and other health benefits, is available in many outlets—health food stores, vitamin shops, grocery stores, health clubs, and more. Coconut water is sold in—bottles, cartons, cans, and even in whole fresh coconuts.

LIQUID AND SOLID COCONUT OIL

One of the distinctive features about coconut oil is its high melting point. If you purchase a bottle of coconut oil in the store, it may appear to be a solid with a pure white color. However, if you put it on your countertop or in your cupboard at home, you may notice in a day or two that it has transformed into a clear liquid. One day it can be liquid and the next it can be solid. There is nothing wrong with the oil; this is normal and natural.

Above 76° F (24° C), coconut oil is a colorless liquid, looking much like any other vegetable oil. Below this temperature, however, it solidifies into a snow white solid. Other fats and oils do this too but at lower temperatures. For example, a cube of butter right out of the refrigerator is hard, yet let it sit out on the countertop on a hot day and it will melt into a puddle. Olive oil does the same thing. At room temperature it is liquid, but if you put it into the refrigerator it transforms into a soft waxy solid. So you can expect coconut oil to change from solid to liquid from day to day depending on the temperature where it is stored. In hot environments, it is almost always liquid; in temperate climates, it is usually solid, especially during the winter months.

You can use the oil for food preparation whether it is in a solid or liquid form. When it is solid, it melts very quickly. Like butter, when you put it in a hot pan or on hot foods, it readily melts. The opposite is also true. If you combine liquid coconut oil with cold foods, the oil will rapidly solidify. For example, if you pour coconut oil over cold foods, it will "freeze" in place. If poured over hot or warm foods, the oil will remain liquid. Animals like it either way, so it really doesn't matter how you serve it to them.

Coconut oil is very heat stable, with a smoke point of about 360° F (182° C), so it makes an excellent cooking and frying oil. Because of its stability, it is slow to oxidize and is resistant to rancidity, with a storage life of about two years—far longer than most other oils. You can use it to fry your foods and refry them again later or pour the drippings onto your pet's food. Because it is very stable, it does not need to be refrigerated and can be stored in the kitchen cupboard.

TYPES OF COCONUT OIL

There are two major types of coconut oil that you will find at the store. One is called "virgin" coconut oil and the other is referred to as "RBD" coconut oil, meaning "refined, bleached, and deodorized." Virgin coconut oil has had minimal processing and retains a delicate coconut aroma and flavor. RBD oil has undergone more extensive processing and all of the flavor and aroma have been removed.

Some people prefer RBD oil because they don't like the taste of coconut or simply don't want all of their foods tasting like coconut. Animals that don't like the taste of virgin coconut oil may take more readily to RBD coconut oil.

I prefer virgin coconut oil myself because I believe that foods are healthiest when they are as close to how they are in nature. The more processing a food undergoes, usually the less healthy it is. However, I sometimes also use RBD oil. While it has undergone more processing, it is not usually made with chemical extracting agents, only heat and filtering. It is still a healthy oil, much healthier than other vegetable oils because it still has the MCFAs. MCFAs are unaffected by the processing. Since coconut oil is heat stable, heat processing does not degrade it. A small amount of some vitamins such as vitamin E may be decreased somewhat, but the main point of giving your pets the oil is not for the vitamins but for the MCFAs. None of the MCFAs are destroyed or harmed in processing. RBD coconut oil contains the same amount of MCFAs as virgin coconut oil.

When you go to the store, you can tell the difference between the two types of coconut oil by the labeling. Virgin coconut oil will always state the word "Virgin" prominently on the label. Sometimes it may even say "Extra Virgin" but that is just another way of indicating that it is a virgin oil. Adding the word "Extra" has no significance other than as a marketing tactic.

Processed coconut oil is rarely ever labeled as being "RBD." Manufacturers usually use some other term such as "Pure," "Organic," or "Expeller Pressed." The key to identifying RBD oil is to look for the word "virgin." If that word is *not* on the label, it means it is RBD regardless of any other terms used.

You can also tell if coconut oil is virgin or RBD by its taste, smell, and appearance. Virgin coconut oil will have a mild coconut flavor and smell and will always be snow white when solid and colorless when liquid. RBD oils will be tasteless and odorless and will be white like virgin coconut oil when solid but either colorless or slightly yellow when liquid, depending on whether they used fresh or sun-dried coconut (copra). Sun-dried coconut tends to produce a yellow tinge to the oil during processing.

Some brands are labeled "Organic." Both virgin and RBD coconut oils can be organic. Legally, to print the word "Organic" on the label, the oil must be certified by a licensed inspector and pass stringent requirements in growing and processing. Certification must be renewed every year. Organic certification is very expensive and most coconut farmers cannot afford it. Organic certification is really not necessary because 95 percent of all the coconut harvested is grown and processed under organic conditions. So the non-organic coconut products you buy in the store are most likely just as organic as the more expensive certified organic products.

I suggest you feed your pet virgin coconut oil because animals generally love the taste. If your pet does not like it, try expeller pressed (RBD) or even coconut milk. If your pet still doesn't take to it, try mixing a little bacon or beef drippings or other animal fat into expeller pressed coconut oil. You don't need a lot of animal fat; a ratio of 1:4 animal fat to coconut oil would be fine. Over time you can gradually reduce the amount of animal fat until you are feeding your pet just coconut oil.

Not all brands of coconut oil taste the same, even if they are virgin. There are many ways to process virgin coconut oil. Consequently, the flavor and aroma will vary some from brand to brand. Some brands have a very nice, delicate coconut aroma and flavor and are very tasty. Others have a strong flavor and might even taste a little smoky, due to processing using open flames. If your pet turns up its nose when offered coconut oil, it may be simply the quality of the oil. Taste it yourself. Does it taste good? Try several brands and use the one that tastes best to you and your pet.

COCONUT MILK

Another product that you should consider feeding to your pet is coconut milk. Coconut milk is rich in fat. This is a good thing. The fats in coconut milk are the same as coconut oil. In fact, coconut oil is often extracted directly from coconut milk. So coconut milk is a good source of MCFAs. A typical 14 ounce (400 ml) can of coconut milk contains about 5 tablespoons of coconut oil. In addition to the MCFAs, it contains proteins, vitamins, and minerals; it has a little carbohydrate but no sugar, making it a healthy food for your pet.

Most mammals love milk. They were all weaned on it. If given the chance, they readily lap it up even as adults. Coconut milk has a rich, creamy taste and texture that animals adore. You can feed them coconut milk straight (I usually dilute it by about half) or you can mix it into their food.

The coconut milk you purchase at the store in cans has been cooked, but some people prefer raw, natural coconut milk. It is healthier and tastier. You can make your own fresh coconut milk from either a fresh mature coconut (the type you can buy at your local grocery store) or from unsweetened, unsulfured, dried flaked or desiccated coconut. See the recipe in Chapter 11.

When buying coconut milk at the store, look for a brand that is unsweetened and free from all preservatives and chemical additives. If the ingredient label lists difficult to pronounce multisyllabic words, buy another brand. While there are some brands of coconut milk that are made from nothing but coconut, most will include at least guar gum if nothing else. Guar gum is a soluble fiber derived from the guar bean and is often used as a thickener in coconut milk and other foods. It is relatively harmless.

Coconut milk spoils quickly, so once you open the can, or make it from scratch, you need to refrigerate it. Freshly made coconut milk (which has not been pasteurized) has a shorter shelf life than the commercially made product. If refrigerated, fresh milk will remain good for about three to four days, while commercially prepared coconut milk will last a few days longer.

Freshly made coconut milk will separate after standing for several hours, the fat floating to the top. This is a natural process and nothing to be afraid of. Simply give the container a shake to mix it before serving. Commercially prepared coconut milk avoids this by adding thickeners that retard separation.

MAINTENANCE AND TREATMENT DOSAGE

You don't want to drop a big blob of coconut oil into your pet's dinner bowl. Although coconut oil is a food and is harmless, it can loosen the bowels if too much is eaten too soon.

A good daily maintenance dose of coconut oil, whether solid or liquid, is 1 teaspoon (5 g) per 10 pounds (4.5 kg) of body weight for carnivorous pets (dogs, cats, ferrets); ⅛ teaspoon (0.6 g) per pound (450 g) for small herbivores (Guinea pigs, hamsters, gerbils, parrots); and ½ teaspoon (2.5 g) per 10 pounds (4.5 kg) for large herbivores (horses, goats, sheep). Give the maintenance dose once daily. You can give it to your pet whole – many like to lick it off the spoon or their owner's fingers – or you can add it to their foods. Most pets readily eat it, but a few are cautious about eating something unfamiliar or will refuse it altogether. If this is the case, mix the

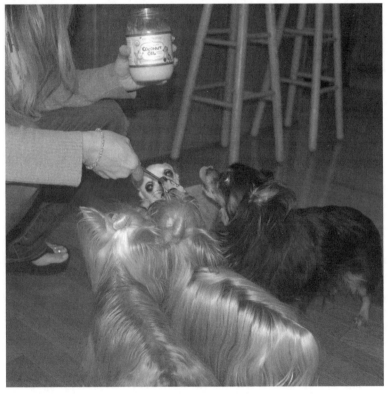

Everybody lining up for their daily dose of coconut oil.

Daily Dose of Coconut Oil

Carnivores and omnivores
1 teaspoon (5g) per 10 pounds (4.5 kg) of body weight
Small herbivores
1/8 teaspoon (0.6 g) per 1 pound (450 g) of body weight
Large herbivores
1/2 teaspoon (2.5 g) per 10 pounds (4.5 kg) of body weight

These are safe daily maintenance doses for most pets, however, you may give a little more or less as you see fit.

melted oil into your pet's food. Over time your pet will gradually become accustomed to the taste and will lap it up by itself.

If your pet has some health issue you are trying to address, you may want to increase the daily dosage to 2 teaspoons (10 g) per 10 pounds (4.5 kg), or twice the maintenance dose. Generally it is best to split this larger dosage in two smaller doses and give it twice daily. Adding the oil to foods reduces the risk of diarrhea. Your pet should adapt to the higher dose within a couple of weeks or so.

When you first introduce your pet to coconut oil, do not start out with these doses, not even the maintenance dose. Most pets will do fine on the maintenance dose; but coconut oil can have lubricating effect on some pets when they first begin to eat it and it may cause frequent urges to go outside or even cause accidents in the house. This is more likely to happen if your pet normally does not have much fat in its diet. Its digestive system isn't geared to handle the added fat and needs some time to adjust to it. Start off with half the maintenance dose for a week or two. This will allow time for your pet's digestive system to adapt to the added fat. If your pet regularly eats a fair amount of fat, then you can start off with the full maintenance dose without worry.

HEALING REACTIONS

In some pets, particularly those with health problems or who are eating poor quality diets, coconut oil can have a dramatic cleansing or detoxifying effect. Because of coconut oil's antibacterial, antiviral, antifungal, and antiparasitic effects, as well as its ability to boost the efficiency of the immune system and increase energy levels and cellular repair, your pet may experience what is known as a cleaning crisis or healing crisis. This is a period of time of intense cleansing and detoxification. It is a common phenomenon in natural medicine and occurs when people or animals do things to improve their health. As their health improves, they reach a point at which their bodies go into a heightened state of cleansing and repair.

The consequence of this period of intense housecleaning is the onset of various symptoms that could be mistaken for an illness or the flu. The body wants to expel dead and dying parasites, yeast, bacteria, and their poisons, as well as toxins that may have been accumulating in the body for years. Symptoms may include diarrhea, vomiting, sinus congestion and discharge, skin breakouts, fatigue, poor appetite, eye and ear discharge, bad breath and body odor (worse than normal), joint pain, and more. Your pet won't experience all these symptoms, usually only one or two. Symptoms may go away after a day or may hang on for a couple of weeks. Once the symptoms are gone, your pet will be happier and healthier than it was before the healing crisis started.

You should let the cleanse run its course; it is a natural process and not an illness. Do not give your pet drugs to treat the symptoms as this will only interfere with the cleansing process and may stop it altogether. Once stopped, the toxins and disease-causing microbes that the healing crisis was trying to remove remain in the body. Don't be afraid of the healing crisis. It is only temporary and your pet will be much better afterwards.

Not all pets will experience a healing crisis when they start eating coconut oil. In fact, most don't. Generally, the symptoms are so mild you won't notice any changes—except afterwards when you see a shinier coat, loss of odor, better skin health, more energy, and improved overall health.

10

Why Our Pets Get Sick

THE MIRACLE MASH

Feeding our pets is easy: we just pull out a bag of dry dog or cat food and dump it in the dish. That's it. No worries about the proper vitamin or mineral content, the right balance of fat, carbohydrate, and protein. That's been done for us in a ready to eat package for your convenience. It makes you wonder what pet owners ever did before there was kibble—the miracle mash. Come to think of it, what did pet owners feed their dogs and cats a century ago, before they had Science Diet and Purina cat chow?

In the old days, pets made due with table scraps, discarded bones and organ meats, fish heads and guts, unused animal skins and hide, milk pale drippings, and anything they could scrounge up or catch. Dogs are natural scavengers and will eat just about anything that is possibly edible. Cats are true carnivores. They love the hunt and are good at it. Cats were often left to fend for themselves, living off of rats, mice, birds, insects, and anything else they could catch. People kept cats specifically to control mice and rats. Back then, people weren't too concerned about their pet's health and the animals had to more or less fend for themselves.

Our pet's wild ancestors ate entirely off the land, not scientifically formulated conglomerations of wheat, soy, and meat by-products. They survived for millions of years on this kind of diet, longer than humans have been around. This is the diet they were designed to eat and to thrive on.

Commercial dog food as we know it didn't exist until the 1960s. Canned pet food has been around for nearly a century, but dry pet food is a more recent creation. The invention of the first commercial dog food is credited to James Spratt, of Cincinnati, Ohio. In the late 1850s, Spratt went to London to sell lightning rods. When his ship arrived, the crew threw their leftover hardtack (hard flour biscuits) onto the dock, where they were gobbled up by hordes of stray dogs. Seeing the dogs eagerly devouring the hardtack gave him the idea for creating the world's first dog biscuit. His recipe was a baked mixture of wheat, beet root, and vegetables bound together with beef blood. When Spratt's Patent Meat Fibrine Dog Cakes came on the market in 1860, the pet-food industry was born. Other companies came out with their own dog biscuits, sparking creative marketing to beat the competition. Some paid veterinarians to endorse their products while others claimed to cure dogs of worms and various diseases. Sounds a lot like the marketing tactics used today. Dog biscuits, however, were more of a treat than a food. They only supplemented the pet's diet of table scraps and whatever else could be found.

Horse meat, bones, and discarded parts of animals from slaughterhouses, which were considered unfit for human consumption, were another source of food for pets in the late 1800s and early 1900s. While this may sound unappetizing to us, raw organ meats, bones, heads, and hoofs are highly nutritious to dogs and cats and are actually very similar to the diet of their wild ancestors.

With the advent of canning technology, slaughterhouse waste was cooked, canned, and marketed as pet food. Canned pet food provided a way to dispose of animal scraps while reaping easy profits. During World War II, however, there was a metal shortage. Tin was rationed for the war effort and tin cans were no longer available for pet foods. Manufacturers were forced to seek new ways to preserve and market pet foods. Drying or dehydrating seemed the most logical direction to head.

By the mid 1950s pet food companies began using a technology borrowed from the cereal industry known as extrusion or kibbling. Thus, kibble was born.

Kibbling is the same process used today to make dry dog and cat food (as well as Froot Loops, Lucky Charms, Cheerios, and other breakfast cereals—or people kibble). It involves taking grains, vegetables, and meat meal and grinding and mashing them together, steaming the mixture at high temperatures, then pushing (or extruding) the mixture through a narrow opening. As the hot, pressurized dough exits the extruder, it is cut into tiny pieces by a set of rapidly whirling knives. As the dough reaches normal air pressure, it expands or puffs into its final shape. This creates the little shapes we know as kibble. The kibble is dried and then sprayed with a mixture of vitamins, minerals, fat, and flavorings to make it more palatable and to meet nutritional requirements.

Dry pet food is made as cheaply as possible to maximize profits. The concern is not about nutrition, but profit. After all, it is *only* pet food. Kibble is composed primarily of cheap grains—fillers that take up room and fill the pet's stomach—with only a token amount of "meat meal" and meat "by-products." Protein content is beefed up using soy and wheat gluten rather than real meat. Flavoring agents and flavor enhancers such as salt and MSG are added to improve the taste and encourage pets to eat it. The nutritional value of kibble straight from the extruder is very poor, so they add a sprinkling of vitamins and minerals to avoid deficiency diseases. Cheap synthetic vitamins are used that have less bioactivity than real vitamins and are often less absorbable but will prevent blatant symptoms of nutritional deficiency disease.

When kibble was first tested, the results were not as expected. Animals that ate it exclusively developed severe nutritional deficiencies, tumorous growths, and other health problems. Obviously, this miracle mash was a nutritional catastrophe. In order to avoid blatant health problems, a required minimum amount of protein, fat, vitamins, and minerals was established. A carbohydrate limit wasn't set because kibble is already overloaded in this substance. Besides, carbohydrate is not even required for the health of dogs or cats.

By adding a certain amount of the various nutrients—protein, fat, vitamins, and minerals—the product can now be labeled as "complete and balanced"—the mark that a dry pet food has met industry standards. Veterinarians endorse it and pet food manufacturers claim it has everything needed to make your dog or cat healthy and, depending on the brand, even boost energy in older pets, restore bad joints, kill worms, and...hey, wait a minute! This sounds an awful lot like the same marketing gimmicks used to sell dog biscuits in the 1800s. And it is! These tactics sold dog biscuits a century ago and they're selling kibble today.

Pet food companies compete against each other, so they use marketing gimmicks to get the edge on their competition. All brands and varieties of kibble are basically the same. They use the same basic ingredients and the same extrusion process. There may be slight variations in the ingredients and minor adjustments to the vitamin and mineral content, but the changes don't amount to anything significant. Kibble is still kibble. However, making these small changes allows manufacturers to market their products to different audiences. You've got kibble for young dogs, kibble for senior dogs or dogs with arthritis, kibble for big dogs and for little dogs, and on and on. If you examine the ingredients closely, although there are some slight differences, you will find they are all pretty much alike.

The nutritional profile in kibble is set by the American Association of Feed Control Organizations (AAFCO). AAFCO guidelines break the components of a healthy diet into four main categories: protein, fat, vitamins, and minerals. In order to advertise and market a product as "complete and balanced," it must supply a minimum amount of each of these. Most varieties of kibble meet these requirements with little variation. Specific ingredients can be added or increased to capture a niche market. For example, adding glucosamine sulfate for joint health or fish oil for brain health. However, the amount of these special substances added usually doesn't amount to anything and would have minimal effect, if any. They are only added as marketing gimmicks.

Adding vitamins and minerals and other gimmicky items to an inherently nutritionally poor food doesn't make the food any healthier. Would adding a few vitamins and minerals to wood pulp make it a health food? Of course not! So, why would kibble be any different? But that is what pet food manufacturers are trying to tell us. They pay veterinarians good money to repeat this mantra. There is much more to food than just vitamins, and minerals. The sugar and carbohydrate content can have a very pronounced impact on health. The type and the amount of fat too, can be extremely important, as well as the source and type of protein. There are half a dozen vitamins that are routinely added to foods, but there are literally thousands of other nutrients, which are not classified as "vitamins" that play important roles in good health, such as beta-carotene, gamma-carotene, lycopene, CQ10, and bioflavonoids. Many of these have important antioxidant properties necessary for achieving and maintaining good health. In addition, there are 60 major and minor minerals that have been identified as playing important roles in cell function. Most pet foods contain only half a dozen or so.

The quality of the protein used is an important issue. Protein is made from amino acids. There are 20 amino acids that are important to in the diet. Of these, nine are considered essential nutrients. Three more are considered conditionally essential, meaning they are essential during different stages of life. From these nine essential and three conditionally essential amino acids, the body can make the remaining amino acids—all of which are necessary to maintain good health. The quality of any particular source of protein is based on how many of the essential and conditionally essential amino acids are present.

A food can be high in protein yet still be a poor protein source because it lacks essential amino acids. Protein in most plant foods is considered incomplete, meaning it lacks some of the essential amino acids. Some plant protein is very deficient. Simply because a plant has protein in it does not mean that the protein it has is as good as another source of protein. For this reason, vegans must combine various plant protein sources to assure they get all the essential amino acids. Meat, eggs, and milk have the highest quality of protein. They have most or all of the essential amino acids in the right ratio and combining with other protein sources is unnecessary. Eggs are the standard by which all other protein sources are compared because they contain 100 percent of the essential and conditionally essential amino acids in the ratio they need to be. They are the ideal protein source.

Commercial pet foods are required to have a certain amount of protein to meet AAFCO standards. However, protein content is not measured but is instead calculated based on nitrogen content.

Protein is roughly 16 percent nitrogen by weight, so the nitrogen levels in food are measured to determine (i.e., estimate) the quantity of protein present. Unfortunately, there are other substances that contain nitrogen, mimicking protein and sometimes adulterating the test results. Protein from soy, grains, gluten, hair, cartilage, gelatin, and other sources boost the nitrogen levels and gives a false impression of the "meat" content.

Adding other nitrogen sources can artificially boost measurable protein content to conform with AAFCO levels. One well publicized example is the Menu Foods fiasco of 2007. Menu Foods, a company that produces dog food for several name brand pet food companies, imported wheat protein (gluten) from China that was tainted with the chemical melamine. Melamine contains 67 percent nitrogen. Visually, wheat flour is indistinguishable from wheat gluten and one could easily be mistaken for the other. Wheat flour tainted with melamine would produce a nitrogen reading consistent with that of gluten, so even a nitrogen analysis would not have shown anything awry. Wheat flour is much cheaper than wheat gluten. If it weren't for one misstep, nobody would have been the wiser. The problem was that melamine is poisonous to dogs and cats. Tainted pet food was sold across the country, resulting in illness and numerous deaths. Over 260 dog and cat food products were recalled, including foods for horses, fish, and reptiles.[1] If it weren't for the deaths, no one probably would have known that these tainted pet foods were protein deficient and they would have continued to be sold to unsuspecting pet owners for years. Makes you wonder what other ingredients may be in our pets' foods to artificially boost nitrogen (protein) readings.

WHAT'S IN YOUR PET'S FOOD?

The photos on the package and in advertisements suggest that pet foods are made from fresh luscious vegetables, healthy whole grains, prime cuts of meat, and milk. In truth, it is a mixture of chemicals, preservatives, rancid fats, rancid meat by-products, rendered meat (dead and sometimes diseased animals), manufactured flavorings and taste enhancers, cheap fillers (soy, corn, oats, wheat), corn syrup...It's enough to make anybody sick, and that's exactly what it is doing to our pets! It's making them sick!

Do you know what's in your dog or cat food? Have you even read the ingredients label? Let's look at an example: Kibbles 'n Bits Original Savory Beef and Chicken Flavor.

> **Ingredients**: corn, soybean meal, beef and bone meal, ground wheat flour, animal fat (BHA used as preservative), corn syrup, wheat middlings, water sufficient for processing, animal digest (source of chicken flavor), propylene glycol, salt, hydrochloric acid, potassium chloride, caramel color, sorbic acid (used as a preservative), sodium carbonate, minerals (ferrous sulfate, zinc oxide, manganous oxide, copper sulfate, calcium iodate, sodium selenite), choline chloride, vitamins (vitamin E supplement, vitamin A supplement, niacin supplement, D-calcium pantothenate, riboflavin supplememnt, pyridoxine hydrochloride, thiamine mononitrate, vitamin D3 supplement, folic acid, biotin, vitamin B12 supplement), calcium sulfate, titanium dioxide, yellow #5, yellow #6, red #40, BHA (used as a preservative), dl methionine.

The ingredients are listed in order of predominance by weight. That means that the product contains more of the first ingredient than any other single ingredient and more of the second ingredient than any other listed afterwards, and so on. The first two ingredients, which comprise the majority of the entire product, are corn and soybean meal. While these products do contribute some to the overall protein content, they are used primary as inexpensive fillers.

We come to meat with the third ingredient—beef and bone meal. What is that? These are rendered products derived from waste animal tissue such as bone, blood, hair, hoof, horn, hide, organs, and believe it or not, manure. Along with the intestines comes the colon and its contents. The majority of animal products comes from slaughterhouse waste but also includes restaurant grease and butcher shop trimmings, expired grocery store meat, and the carcasses of euthanized and dead animals. All of these unwanted animal parts are boiled together and ground into a meat and bone meal. Some brands may claim to include "fresh" meat, but none of the meat products in kibble are fresh. Think about it. How can fresh meat remain fresh in a dried product? It's just a marketing tactic.

What is rendering? Raw materials are dumped into large vat and boiled for several hours. Rendering separates fat, removes water, and kills bacteria, and other organisms. However, the high temperatures used (270°F/130°C) destroys enzymes and alters the natural fats and proteins found in the raw ingredients.

Because of persistent rumors that rendered by-products contain dead dogs and cats, the FDA conducted a study looking for the drug pentobarbital (used to put animals down) in pet foods. They found it. Ingredients that were most commonly associated with the presence of pentobarbital were meat and bone meal and animal fat. However, when they looked for canine and feline DNA, none was found. Euthanized pets and roadkill were used in pet food in the past. While there are no laws against it, today pet food companies deny that their products contain any such materials. So why did the FDA find pentobarbital in the pet foods they analyzed? Perhaps it came from farm animals that were put down. So-called "4D" animals (dead, dying, diseased, disabled) were only recently banned for human consumption but are still legitimate ingredients for pet food. Regardless of the source, a drug used to kill animals shouldn't be in pet food.

The fourth ingredient is wheat flour, another filler. The next ingredient is animal fat, which is separated from the meat and bone meal during the rendering process. Various fats are used in pet foods—animal fat, canola oil, sunflower oil, soybean oil, and so on. The biggest problem with these fats is that they are all rancid, every last one of them. When vegetable oils and even animal fats are exposed to heat, light, and oxygen, they oxidize, that is, go rancid. These oils are exposed to heat, light, and oxygen from the very start in the kibbling process. Rancidity begins in the factory and continues as the product is packed, shipped, stored, and placed on store shelves waiting to be sold. It could be months old by the time it is sold and used.

As you recall from Chapter 2, rancid fat produces destructive molecules known as free radicals. Free radicals are associated with all forms of degenerative disease. They break down tissues and damage cells.

Next on the list is corn syrup, which is added to sweeten the kibble and make it more palatable. Does your dog or cat really need sugar in its diet? Sugar has now been linked to a number of degenerative diseases in humans such as gum disease, Alzheimer's, and diabetes. It is just as bad, and probably even worse, for our pets.

The next ingredient, wheat middlings, may sound wholesome but it is actually the waste produced from wheat milling—the wheat dust and floor sweepings. It is just another cheap filler. Animal digest is a flavoring sprayed on the kibble after it's been cooked to improve its taste so that animals will eat it. Salt is also added to enhance the flavor and palatability.

Propylene glycol is a chemical used to sustain the dryness of the kibble—to keep it from becoming soggy in the package. It also acts as a preservative because moisture promotes bacterial and fungal growth. While it is approved for use in dog food, it is banned from cat food because it is has been linked blood disorders and anemia.

Caramel color and chemical dyes like yellow #5, yellow #6, and red #40 are totally unnecessary. They serve no purpose except to make the kibble appeasing to the people who buy it. Many artificial coloring agents have been linked to cancer and other health issues.

There is a smattering of a few other chemicals and preservatives (sorbic acid and BHA), along with the token vitamins and minerals that make the kibble "complete and balanced," and therefore, approved by veterinarians everywhere.

The last ingredient is dl methionine, one of the essential amino acids. This is interesting. If the protein in meat contains amino acids, why is a methionine supplement added? It is added for the same reason all the vitamins and minerals are added—to compensate for a nutritionally poor product. If kibble contained real food, it wouldn't need these supplements. When a cat eats a mouse, it doesn't need a vitamin, mineral, and amino acid supplement to go along with it. It gets all of the nutrition it needs from the mouse. Cats can and do live long happy lives eating nothing but rodents and insects. Meat is a good source of methionine, but there is so little real meat in kibble, and plant proteins are such poor sources, that methionine must be added to prevent nutritional deficiencies. After looking at all of these ingredients is it any wonder why our pets are getting sick?

Don't be deceived into thinking canned pet foods are any better. They contain the same basic ingredients as kibble. Although those little chunks of "meat" look meaty, they are composed mostly of grains and wheat gluten and are molded into their shapes and suspended in gelatin to look like meat. It's essentially canned kibble. The water content is the main difference. Canned pet food contains about 75 percent water; kibble has only 10 percent.

ARE PETS HEALTHIER TODAY?

You might think that because your veterinarian recommends these foods, they are the best for your pet. Think again. Veterinarians are trained to believe that the "scientifically" formulated canned and kibbled foods are the best foods for your pet simply because they are "complete and balanced." Pet food companies invest a lot of money into beating this concept into their heads. Veterinarians are taught this in school and come out believing it. In addition, the relationship between veterinarians and pet food companies is similar to that between doctors and pharmaceutical companies. While veterinarians seek to provide a needed service, the main goal of pet food companies is to make money. If they can convince veterinarians that their food is the best, they make more money from the veterinarians' promotion. Much of the continued education on nutrition and diet that veterinarians receive comes from pet food companies – a source with an agenda and riddled with marketing propaganda.

"It is hard to believe that dedicated animal healers—veterinary surgeons—will recommend commercial pet food," says Dr. Ian Billinghurst, the creator of the BARF (Biologically Appropriate Raw Food) diet. "I find this hard to believe because as a practicing veterinary surgeon, I constantly see the enormous difference in health between pets raised on commercial pet food compared to those raised on a biologically appropriate raw food diet. I see the enormous change for good in the health of pets switched from cooked to a raw whole food diet. Despite that very obvious connection between commercial pet food and the poor health of the animals consuming it, commercial pet food has become the accepted way to feed pets throughout the civilized world!"

Kibble is promoted as all that our pets need to be healthy. We are advised not to feed them table scraps. Real meat and vegetables aren't good for them, we're told. They need kibble, because it's "complete and balanced." Table scraps might be "unbalanced" and that could be bad for your pet. Or it might upset the animal's delicate stomach. How did the animal's stomach get so delicate that it can't handle a piece of steak? Our pet's ancestors ate the bones, brains, guts, skin, and hair of prey animals. They even ate rotting meat and insects. Why were their stomachs able to handle this disgusting menagerie but our modern pets can't handle a simple piece of meat? Could it be the kibble that is at fault, making their stomachs unable to handle real foods?

Kibble is really no different from Froot Loops breakfast cereal. Look at the ingredient label. Like kibble, the main ingredients are grains (corn, wheat, and oats) accompanied by vegetable oil (partially hydrogenated at that), sugar and salt, flavorings and colorings, preservatives (BHT), and a smattering of synthetic vitamins and minerals. Served with pasteurized milk you get a few more vitamins and minerals, protein, and some fat. It is pretty much the nutritional equivalent of kibble. Can you imagine living your entire life eating nothing but Froot Loops day after day, year after year, on and on until you die? How would that affect your health? You would be lucky to survive 10 or 15 years, and so would your pet eating kibble. Actually, you probably wouldn't survive for long. You would likely develop any number of degenerative conditions, just like our pets are experiencing today. The ingredients in Froot Loops are:

Ingredients: sugar, whole grain corn flour, wheat flour, whole grain oat flour, oat fiber, soluble corn fiber, partially hydrogenated vegetable oil, salt, sodium ascorbate and ascorbic acid (vitamin C), niacinamide, reduced iron, natural orange lemon, cherry, raspberry blueberry, lime and other natural flavors, red #40, blue #2, turmeric color, yellow #6, zinc oxide, annatto color, blue #1, pyridoxine hydrochloride (vitamin B6), Riboflavin (vitamin B2), Thiamin hydrochloride (vitamin B1) Vitamin A palmitate, BHT, Folic Acid, Vitamin D, Vitamin B12.

Back in the day, pets did not suffer from all the degenerative conditions that they do now. Occasionally a pet would get cancer or some stomach troubles, but it was the exception, not the rule. Today, it seems like all dogs and cats suffer from degenerative disease of one type or another. For example, by the age of 10 or 11 approximately half of dogs show signs of dementia. Dementia is not a part of the normal aging process, it is a disease caused primary by a poor diet. The same is true for arthritis, cancer, Crohn's disease, colitis, dental cavities, gum disease, allergies, and others, all of which our pets are increasingly being plagued with.

Oh, but kibble-fed dogs and cats live long lives up to 15 to 20 years, we are told. They are living longer now than they used to, so old age is bound to bring with it some health problems. Again disease is not the same as old age. Just because a dog is old does not mean he is destined to develop cancer or dementia or colitis. These diseases are caused by something in their environment, regardless of their age. Dogs can live long, full lives without ever experiencing the degenerative diseases kibble fed dogs do. And live just as long if not longer.

There have been no studies on longevity in dogs before we had kibble, so no direct comparisons can be made. However, there are records of dogs living off of table scraps and whatever else they could find. The world record for dog longevity was reported in 1939 (long before kibble was around). An Australian cattle dog named Bluey died in 1939 at the age of 29 years. That's the equivalent to 203 human years! Talk about longevity! Bluey's longevity record is documented by *The Guinness Book of World Records*.[2]

In 2004, Jerry, a cattle dog-bull terrier cross, was reported by his veterinarian to be 27 years old, the equivalent of 198 years for a human. By now, Jerry may have broken Bluey's longevity record; I don't have the details. But Jerry, like Bluey, never tasted kibble. He lived with an Australian Aboriginal family in Australia's Outback eating table scraps and whatever else he could catch or find. Like Bluey, he didn't suffer from arthritis or dementia but was active even into his old age.

Bluey and Jerry are not isolated incidents. Another dog, Teddy, a poodle born in 1908 in New Orleans, also lived to be 29. Again this was before kibble.[3] Adjutant, a black Labrador living in England, was reported by *The Guinness Book of World Records* as being born in 1936, also prior to kibble. He died in 1963 at the age of 27 years.[4] There are apparently many non-kibble fed dogs that have lived very long lives without the disease and suffering that kibble-fed dogs experience.

Dogs and cats existed for millions of years eating raw meat. They did not have the common ailments that afflict a lot of modern day dogs and cats because they ate the way Mother Nature intended. Now our animals are fed corn, soy meal, rancid oils, sugar, and chemicals. It's no wonder they have so many health problems.

There is power in eating raw foods. Getting back to a natural diet can reverse many of our pets' common health problems. Even just a little raw food can have an impact on the health of your pet. "I've been joking for awhile that I thought my kitty, Thor, might be suffering kitty dementia or Alzheimer's," says J. C. "A concept that once seemed amusing has just become sad, because it's true. I didn't think it possible, not sure why, but I recognize the behavior and the look in his eyes very well after caring for my grandmother with Alzheimer's for many years. He's so forlorn and needy, it's like having a newborn baby in the house. My sons and I noticed he was *perfectly* normal for two whole weeks after catching (and eating) a rat! Ordinarily I would have taken it from him and not allowed him to eat it, but he snuck it in and left only the ears as evidence. Pretty gross, but I wonder what nutrients he got from eating a rat that seemed to be a cure-all for two entire weeks!" The rat was not only raw, but was eaten whole, skin, bones, guts, stomach, and all.

Our pet's growing incidence of ill health has mirrored our own as our diet has changed over the past century from fresh farm produce, meat, and dairy to canned, packaged, frozen, and processed foods. Before the turn of the 20th century, when modern food processing was invented, degenerative disease was uncommon. Back then, heart disease was unheard of, cancer was rare, Alzheimer's wasn't even recognized, and diabetes was essentially nonexistent. These so-called diseases of modern civilization didn't appear to any great extent until after modern food processing was introduced in the early 1900s. Age and lifespan have nothing to do with it. People a century ago were living into their 90s and beyond, like they do now, but they didn't suffer as much as we do now. People today are suffering from degenerative or "old age" diseases at younger and younger ages. Diabetes, cancer, and even Alzheimer's are affecting people in their

20s, 30s, and 40s. Advancing age doesn't cause these diseases; diet and lifestyle do.

When people lived naturally, eating what they were able to catch, grow, or pick, they were much healthier. This observation has been proven time and time again. It is just as true for our pets as it is for us.

NUTRITION AND PHYSICAL DEGENERATION

The link between the rise of degenerative disease and diet was clearly demonstrated back in the 1930s by Weston A. Price, DDS (1870-1948). Dr. Price served as Chairman of the Research Section of the American Dental Association from 1914-1923 and is noted for his extensive research on nutrition and dental health.

During his long career as a practicing dentist, he observed an increasing incidence of tooth decay and dental deformities and other health problems late in his career that were rare in his earlier years. He was seeing more and more children with narrow dental arches and crowded teeth. When the wisdom teeth came in, there often wasn't room for them, which required that they be extracted. This was a curious phenomenon because early in his career patients rarely had to have wisdom teeth removed. This deformity of the jaw appeared to be a modern phenomena. Remains of ancient humans showed broad dental arches and healthy wisdom teeth. It didn't make sense that the human body, as perfectly designed as it is, would suddenly grow teeth that didn't work and required surgical removal. At no time in the history of the human race had there been a need to remove wisdom teeth from so many people. It wasn't just the teeth; he noticed that the general health of his patients was declining. They were developing degenerative diseases at an increasing rate. He was seeing the so-called diseases of "old age" in younger and younger patients.

Price was a first-hand witness to the transformation and revolution of modern food processing. In his lifetime he witnessed the change from eating primarily fresh foods to eating commercially prepared, packaged foods. He wondered if the changes in the diet were related to the decline in health, and set out to find the answer.

The way he planned to do this was to compare the health of people who ate traditional diets with those who ate modern processed foods. To avoid other influences that may affect health, he compared people of the same genetic background who lived in the same geographic area. The only difference would be their diets.

Today it is nearly impossible to find populations that rely solely on traditional foods. Modern foods are found virtually everywhere throughout the world. But in the 1930s there were still many populations that subsisted primarily on their ancestral foods without modern influences.

Dr. Price spent nearly a decade traveling around the world locating and studying these populations. He traveled to isolated valleys in the Swiss Alps, the Outer and Inner Hebrides off the coast of Scotland, visited Eskimo villages in Alaska, American Indians in central and northern Canada, the Melanesians and Polynesians on numerous islands throughout the South Pacific, tribes in eastern and central Africa, the Aborigines of Australia, Malay tribes on islands north of Australia, the Maori of New Zealand, and South American Indians in Peru and the Amazon Basin.

When Dr. Price visited an area, he would examine the people's health, particularly their teeth, and make careful note of the foods they ate and meticulously analyzed the nutritional content of the diet. Samples of the foods were sent to his laboratory where detailed analyses were made. It didn't take long for him to notice the contrast in health between those who lived entirely on indigenous foods and those who had incorporated modern foods into their diets.

Wherever he found people living on traditional foods, he noted that both their dental and physical health were in excellent condition, but when the people began eating modern processed foods, their health quickly declined. In the absence of modern medical care, physical degeneration was pronounced. Dental diseases, as well as infectious and degenerative diseases such as arthritis and tuberculosis, were common among those eating modern foods.

He also found that it didn't take a dramatic change in the diet for degenerative disease to begin to creep in. Simply adding a few commercial products, which displaced more nutritious foods, was all that was needed. The most common imported foods were white flour, sugar, processed vegetable oils, and canned meats.

He observed that parents who began adding these modern foods into their diets gave birth to children whose teeth and bone structure was suboptimal. The dental arch became narrowed, teeth became crowded, and wisdom teeth became impacted. In contrast, those parents who ate traditional foods had children with excellent dental health and development. The children possessed wide dental arches, had straight healthy teeth, and wisdom teeth came in without problem. Allergies, too, were completely unknown to the isolated peoples eating traditional diets.

The same degeneration in health that was occurring in these primitive societies when they adopted modern foods was the same that he had been seeing in his dental practice in Ohio. The connection was obvious. Modern processed foods were nutritionally deficient, and as a consequence, people were developing a greater number of degenerative conditions and children were being born with developmental deficiencies. In every single population he studied, regardless of what part of the world, the pattern was the same. There were no exceptions. Dr. Price's findings were published in 1939 in a book titled *Nutrition and Physical Degeneration*. This book, which is still in print, is considered a classic in nutritional science.

Degenerative diseases such as gum disease, heart disease, cancer, asthma, bronchitis, diabetes, arthritis, and allergies are referred to as "diseases of modern civilization." These conditions are rare among primitive societies who live on traditional diets consisting of whole, natural foods. When populations are introduced to modern civilization and adopt processed foods, diseases of modern civilization begin to develop. Dr. Price found that within just a single generation these cultures experienced all of these degenerative conditions, clearly indicating that they are not caused by genetics.

Dr. Price noticed that poor dental health also indicated poor overall health. When people's diets started to include more processed, prepared foods (sugar, white flour, canned meats) it was clearly evident in the condition of their teeth and gums. The same is true for our pets. By the age of three years, all dogs that are raised on commercial pet foods have dental problems.[5]

Proponents of dry pet foods often tell us that kibble is good for pets because it cleans their teeth. The dry, crunchy kibble supposedly scrapes their teeth clean. This is a myth. Kibble cleans an animal's teeth no more than eating dry Froot Loops cleans your kid's teeth. They are both loaded with carbohydrates—the one thing that promotes tooth decay more than anything else! The shearing action from chewing on bones is what cleans the teeth.

Dr. Price never saw people living on natural foods that were overweight. Being overweight is another indicator of poor health. In addition, 40 percent of all dogs in the US today are overweight.[6] Today approximately 90 percent of Americans have some level of dental decay and 65 percent are overweight. Heart disease, high blood pressure, osteoporosis, diabetes, cancer, Alzheimer's, and other diseases of civilization are rampant. Our pets now suffer from these same conditions.

POTTENGER'S CATS

Dr. Price discovered that our diet not only affects our own health, but affects the health of our unborn children far more than you might imagine. In fact, the health problems you may be experiencing now could be a direct result of your parent's diet. The health of your mother, and to a lesser extent your father, sets the stage for how healthy you will be throughout your life and how susceptible you will be to food and environmental allergies and to degenerative disease. A woman's nutrition prior to and throughout pregnancy is crucial to her health and to the growth, development, and health of the infant she conceives. The foods she eats and her level of health not only affect the health of her children, but also her grandchildren.[7]

This is also true for animals as well. A fascinating study with cats and how their health and the health of their offspring was affected by diet was conducted by Francis M. Pottenger, Jr., MD (1901-1967) and colleagues over a ten year period from 1932-1942.

Dr. Pottenger used hormonal extracts from the adrenal cortex of cows and pigs as supplements to treat patients with hormonal problems. At the time, there was no procedure for standardizing hormonal extracts, so manufacturers of these extracts had to use animals, such as cats, to determine potency. The adrenal glands of cats were removed. Without the glands, the cats would die. The dose of adrenal extract required to keep them alive calibrated the level of the extract's potency that could then be used in treating patients.

A number of cats were kept in the hospital laboratory for this purpose. The animals were fed raw milk and cooked meat scraps obtained from the hospital kitchen, including liver, tripe, sweetbreads, brains, heart, and muscle. This diet was considered by the experts of the day to be rich in all the important nutrients. Yet there was a high death rate among the cats after undergoing the surgery, which perplexed Dr. Pottenger. He began noticing that the cats that had been in the laboratory for some time showed signs of nutritional deficiency. All showed a decrease in their reproductive capacity and many of the kittens born in the laboratory had skeletal deformities and organ malfunctions.

Most of the cats were donated to the hospital by local residents. As the cat population increased, the demand for meat scraps exceeded their supply. Pottenger began ordering *raw* meat scraps (organ and muscle meats with bones) from a local meat packing plant. These raw meat scraps were fed to a segregated group of cats and within a few months this group appeared in better health than the animals being fed cooked meat scraps. Their kittens appeared more vigorous, and their survival rate after surgery increased markedly.

This prompted Pottenger to undertake a controlled experiment. What he had observed by chance he wanted to repeat by design. The cats in the Pottenger Cat Study were kept in large outdoor pens and were cared for daily. Each cat was identified and its health and diet was carefully monitored throughout its life. Over the course of ten years Pottenger recorded complete health histories of hundreds of cats used in the study.

The cats were separated into various groups. One group received ⅔ raw meat, ⅓ raw cow's milk, supplemented with cod liver oil (100 percent raw foods). A second group received ⅔ cooked meat, ⅓ raw cow's milk, supplemented with cod liver oil (⅔ cooked and ⅓ raw).

In the raw food group, Pottenger observed that the animals maintained good health throughout their lives. From one generation to the next, they maintained a broad face with broad dental arches, adequate nasal cavities, and healthy teeth. Each sex maintained its distinct anatomical features with the female skull distinctly different from the male. Their membranes were firm and of good color with no evidence of infection or degenerative change. Tissue tone was excellent and the fur of good quality. The calcium and phosphorus content of their bones remained consistent and their internal organs showed full development and normal function. During their lives, they proved resistant to infection, to fleas, and to various other parasites, and they showed no signs of allergies. In general, they were friendly and predictable in their behavior. These cats reproduced one homogeneous generation after another with the average weight of the kittens at birth being 119 grams. Miscarriages were rare and the litters averaged five kittens with the mother cat nursing her young without difficulty.

In the cooked food group, each kitten in a litter was different in size and skeletal pattern. Evidence of deficiency was plainly evident in the narrowed structure of their faces and in the misalignment of their teeth. The bones became weaker and contained less calcium. Heart problems; nearsightedness and farsightedness; underactivity of the thyroid gland; infections of the kidney, liver, testes, ovaries, and bladder; arthritis and inflammation of the joints; and inflammation of the nervous system with paralysis and meningitis all occurred commonly in the cooked meat fed cats. Cooked meat fed cats showed much more irritability. Some females were even dangerous to handle. Intestinal parasites and fleas abounded. Skin lesions and allergies appeared frequently and were progressively worse from one generation to the next. The birth rate was lower among the cooked meat fed cats. Autopsies showed that females frequently had ovarian atrophy and uterine congestion, and the males often had a decreased ability to produce sperm. Spontaneous abortion was common, running about 25 percent in the first deficient generation to about 70 percent in the second generation. Deliveries were generally difficult with many females dying in labor. The mortality rate of the kittens was also high. Following delivery, a few mother cats steadily declined in health only to die from some obscure physiological difficulty. The average weight of the kittens born of cooked meat fed mothers was 100 grams, 19 grams less than the raw meat nurtured kittens. By the third deficient generation, the cats were so physiologically bankrupt that none survived beyond the sixth month of life, thereby terminating the strain.

Dr. Pottenger experimented with other similar diets. Another group received a diet of ⅔ raw milk and ⅓ raw meat. Another group received mostly pasteurized milk and a little raw meat. Again, the

100 percent raw food diet produced healthy cats generation after generation, while the pasteurized milk diet produced cats suffering from multiple deficiency diseases. It is interesting to note that the cooked diets also included some raw food as well, so the diets were not 100 percent cooked. Therefore, having a little raw or fully nutritious food in the diet did not compensate for the rest of nutritional deficiencies in the diet. Dr. Pottenger's cat experiment is described in detail in the book *Pottenger's Cats: A Study in Nutrition* (published by the Price-Pottenger Nutrition Foundation).

It doesn't take a genius to see the obvious similarities between what happened to Pottenger's cats and what is happening to our pets today. Kibble, as well as canned pet food, is always cooked. It is no wonder when it was first given to animals that it caused severe nutritional deficiencies. The addition of a few vitamins and minerals has prevented immediate health problems but has only delayed the inevitable onset of degenerative disease, dental problems, allergies, and other health problems.

11

Foods for Better Health

Adding coconut oil and other coconut products into your pet's diet can bring about remarkable changes for the better in your pet's health. It can boost your pet's immune function, helping it fight off infections and disease and in many cases easing longstanding health issues that have not responded to conventional treatments. Coconut oil is completely safe to eat and to apply on the skin. Many of the beneficial effects obtained from coconut occur because the oil assists or boosts the body's own natural healing functions. The effectiveness of the oil in treating health problems is greatly affected by your pet's diet. If you provide the right materials for repairing and rebuilding bones, muscles, and tissues, healing is enhanced. On the other hand, if your pet is malnourished or fed inappropriate foods, rancid fats, and chemical additives, the healing effects of coconut oil will be limited. In this chapter we will explore how to enhance the healing effects of coconut oil by improving your pet's diet.

WHAT DIET IS THE HEALTHIEST?

The healthiest diet for your pet is one that is species appropriate, that is, one that mimics the diet the animal would eat naturally in the wild. Herbivorous (vegetarian) pets such as rabbits, guinea pigs, hamsters, gerbils, and parrots thrive on plant foods—grass, seeds, nuts, fruit, vegetables, and the like. Omnivores, which eat both plant and animal foods, do best on a mixed diet. Carnivores such as dogs, cats, and ferrets, thrive on a meat based diet. Herbivores and omnivores are relatively easy to feed using commercially prepared plant foods and fresh produce. Carnivores are a different matter. As seen in the previous chapter, commercially made foods for dogs and cats, especially dried foods, are deplorable and are in no way similar to what they would naturally eat in the wild.

Dogs, cats, and ferrets need a good source of quality protein and fat with adequate moisture, supplemented with just a little vegetable or plant material. Although cats, dogs, and ferrets are carnivores, they do eat some plants from the digestive tract of their prey. For optimal health, a mostly raw food, meat based, low-carb diet is the most natural and the healthiest. They are not meant to live on high-carbohydrate or starchy foods such as wheat, corn, rice and soy that are used so abundantly in processed pet foods. These are not their natural foods and they have no need for them. In fact, eating too much starchy foods can cause many health problems, especially blood sugar problems that can promote diabetes, heart and circulation problems, dementia, premature aging, and others.

A relatively high moisture content in the food is also important. A natural diet consists of about 70 percent water, which comes from eating mice, birds, and other small animals. Dry pet foods, such as kibble, contain less than 12 percent moisture. Animals that live on a diet of dried food exist in a state chronic dehydration, which can lead to many health problems over time, especially kidney and skin problems. This is a greater issue with cats and ferrets than it is for dogs, because dogs will drink water when thirsty, but cats and ferrets get most of their water from their foods.

There are many choices of pet food on the market. Some are much better than others. Some are downright awful. They all use fancy terms and marking gimmicks like "All Natural," "Balanced," "Made with Real Meat," and so forth. Which ones are truly the best and which ones should you avoid? Below is a ranking from 1 to 7 of the best to worst foods for dogs, cats, and ferrets.

Don't feel bad if you are not feeding your pet the highest quality foods. Some people do not have the finances, time, or resources to feed their pets the best possible foods. Do what you can. If you can move up the list even a little bit, that is better than doing nothing at all.

#1 Raw Homemade

A balanced, raw, homemade diet is the best quality food for your dog, cat, or ferret. With homemade foods, you know exactly the quality and the types of ingredients you are feeding to your pet. The best foods for your dog or cat would be the same or similar to the types of foods they would get in the wild. Cats and ferrets are primarily carnivores and do best on a diet of mostly raw meaty foods. Dogs are scavengers and do well with raw meats supplemented with some plant foods. Their diets should not be based on cooked grains and soy.

Veterinarians often speak of the importance of getting a "balanced diet." This means getting the appropriate amount of protein, fat, vitamins, minerals, and other nutrients. Eating whole prey animals supplies a complete and balanced diet. Eating table scraps may not. This is one of the reasons why veterinarians don't recommend that pets eat people food. Another reason is that most table scraps are not nutritionally balanced and are usually loaded with nutritionless additives like sugar, starch, MSG, nitrates, dyes, chemical preservatives and such—foods that are not much better than kibble.

Ideally, the food should mimic the same balance and type of ingredients consumed by your pet's wild ancestors. This would include muscle meats, bones, fat, and a variety of organ meats, as well as some vegetable materials. Even strict carnivores eat some plant foods, primarily from the contents of their prey's stomach. Keep in mind that you are mimicking a wild diet, not duplicating it. It is impractical to feed your pet whole animal carcasses. What you want to do is feed your pet foods that supply the same types of nutrients.

Keep the diet varied; use different meats, different organs, and different vegetables. Use fat liberally. Using a mix of ingredients will guarantee a variety of nutrients so that the diet is truly complete and balanced. The contents of a prey animal's stomach provides a great deal of nutrition; see the recipe for stomach stew in the next chapter.

Don't skimp on the fat. Animals love fat and will eat as much as they can get, and for good reason: it is an essential nutrient in their diets. Fat provides far more than just calories. It is necessary for the proper absorption of a variety of nutrients. The best fats for your pet are animal fats, coconut oil, and red palm oil. Olive oil is fine too, but I recommend you avoid most other vegetable oils. Processed vegetable oils are partially rancid when you buy them.

Raw eggs are very nutritious. They are loaded with important vitamins and minerals, supply essential fatty acids, including the harder to get omega 3 fatty acids, and contain the highest quality protein. Pets love the taste. Use them often, preferably free-range or organic eggs.

Making pet food at home can be challenging and time consuming, especially if you are new at it. For starters, I recommend the hearty meat and vegetable stew, or stomach stew as I call it, described in the next chapter. For additional helpful advice, I recommend the book *Real Food for Healthy Dogs and Cats* by Karen Becker, DVM.

#2 Commercial Raw Foods

Some people just don't have the time or inclination to make their own pet food. The next best choice is commercially prepared raw pet foods. These foods save you the time of mixing and matching the various ingredients to get a balanced diet. Since the food is raw, they are kept frozen and stored in the freezer compartment at the store. Not all pet stores have freezers or sell these types of products. You are most likely to find them in small pet shops where the owners know and understand the importance of good pet nutrition. You are less likely to find them at the mega pet stores like PetSmart or Petco.

There are many different brands and varieties. They should contain a variety of ingredients that supply a pet's nutritional needs, including organ meats. Look for the AAFCO label guarantee so you know it has been approved by the American Association of Feed Control Officials as nutritionally "complete and balanced." The "complete and balanced" designation here is more meaningful than it is with dry pet food because the nutrients come from real foods and not synthetic vitamins and chemicals.

One popular raw food brand is BARF (Biologically Appropriate Raw Food). The ingredients in their frozen beef patties are: beef, finely ground beef/pork bone, beef liver, beef kidney, egg, broccoli, celery, spinach, carrot, beef tripe, ground flax seed, dehydrated alfalfa meal, apple, pear, grapefruit, orange, dried kelp, cayenne pepper, cod liver oil, garlic vitamin E, zinc oxide, manganous oxide.

#3 Dehydrated or Freeze-Dried Raw Foods

An option to frozen raw foods is dehydrated or freeze-dried raw foods. You add enough water to reconstitute it to match the 70 percent or so found in natural non-dehydrated raw foods.

The food is dried at low temperatures or, in the case of freeze-dried food, at temperatures below freezing, so it is still raw and retains most of its nutritional value. It is in powder form and when water is added it turns into a thick mush.

This is a good choice for pet owners who want to get off dry or canned foods but don't feel comfortable with fresh or frozen raw foods. It can also be used as a transition food from kibble to raw food if you don't want to feed your pet canned foods.

These products will have a mixture of meat, vegetables, and fruit. An example from one commercial product is dehydrated turkey, potatoes, celery, spinach, carrots, coconut, apples, kelp, eggs, and banana. Note that there are no grains, but there is starch from the potato.

#4 Real Meat Canned Food

If you can't feed your pet any of the raw foods listed above, the next best choice is canned food using real meat, not meat by-products. Look at the ingredient label. Remember, the order of the ingredients is important. Are the first things listed specific name meats, such as beef, chicken, or salmon, or is it meat by-products (unnamed animal protein) or grains? It should be mostly meat and some vegetables; if there are grains, they should be whole grains like wheat flour or brown rice and should be farther down the list. Canned foods contain between 70-80 percent water, similar to that of natural raw foods. Even though canned foods are cooked, they are still healthier than dry food.

Whole meat, such as white chicken meat or salmon, should be the first ingredient followed by water, although sometimes water may the first ingredient. The remaining ingredients may include additional meat, meat by-products, various vegetables, and finally vitamins and minerals. For example, Spot's Stew, chicken flavor, by Halo contains in order: chicken broth, chicken, chicken liver, carrots, celery, zucchini, yellow squash, pasta, green peas, green beans, turkey, barley, rolled oats, various vitamins and minerals. The liquid is chicken broth rather than just water followed by meat and vegetables. There is a little pasta (made from wheat flour and egg whites) and minor amounts of barley and oats. There are no artificial flavorings or chemical additives. All-in-all, it is a fairly good choice for a canned product.

#5 Regular Canned Food

This is canned food made using meat by-products, often in a gelatin base to give it the appearance of real meat. The chunks of meat are formed in a process similar to that in which kibble is made. This is basically kibble in a can. The advantage this product has over dry kibble is that it contains about 70 percent water, providing needed liquids.

A so-called "meaty" chicken dinner from one of the major dog food producers lists the ingredients as: sufficient water for processing, poultry by-products, chicken, animal liver, meat by-products, brewers rice, minerals, sodium tripolyphosphate, vegetable oil, carrageenan, vitamins, xanthan gum, taurine, dried yam, natural flavor, salt, guar gum, marigold extract. The meat is primarily poultry and meat by-products with a little chicken and "animal" liver. Animal liver is rather nebulous term and could have come from anything. The fillers are rice along with carrageenan, xanthan gum, and guar gum, which are thickeners used to thicken the water and make the product appear more substantial than it actually is. The only vegetable is a little dried yam near the bottom of the list. The remaining ingredients are mostly vitamins and minerals, flavor enhancers, and preservatives.

#6 Kibble

Although dry pet food can be labeled as "complete and balanced," it is one of the worst choices for your pet. As described in the previous chapter, it is made from rendered animal carcasses and slaughterhouse and butcher shop wastes, loaded with grain-based fillers, rancid fats, syrup, flavor enhancers, chemical dyes, preservatives, and other questionable additives. It is regarded as nutritionally complete because of the synthetic vitamins and minerals that are added.

Some brands are slightly better than others. The higher quality kibble is made from fish, beef, or chicken meal instead of meat by-products. Meal is made from meat that has been dried and ground up.

The better products will contain grains or soy. However they will contain other sources of starch such as white potatoes, sweet potatoes, peas, and such. Starch is needed for the extrusion process in making kibble. Simply because it is grain free, does not make it carbohydrate free.

They will always contain some type of fat or oil, which will be terribly rancid. Whether it is vegetable oil, animal fat, or fish oil, it will all be rancid.

#7 Semi-Moist Pouched Food

This is a moist or softer version of kibble. It has all the bad things kibble has going for it and in some cases an added ingredient called propylene glycol—a chemical very similar to ethylene glycol (antifreeze). Ethylene glycol is poisonous to humans and pets and while propylene glycol is considered safer, it isn't something you want to be feeding to your pets. It has been banned from cat foods because of its toxicity, but is still used in some dog and other pet foods. Since this product is moist, it is vulnerable to bacterial and fungal growth, so it must contain significantly more preservatives than dried foods to prevent spoilage. These chemicals are not food and can be toxic, which is why bacteria and fungi can't grow in their presence.

IS RAW MEAT SAFE?

The biggest fear people have about feeding their pets raw foods is that it will make them sick. We often hear about the dangers of people eating raw or undercooked meat. Food poisoning scares appear in the news all the time. This happens when Salmonella, E. coli, and other potentially harmful bacteria contaminate raw food, whether it is meat, vegetables, or fruit. But this danger is to humans, not dogs and cats.

Our pet's wild ancestors thrived on a diet of raw meat. They never ate cooked meat or kibble and never worried about the bacteria that might be on their prey's skin or hair or in its stomach, intestine, colon, or their contents. Dogs and other scavengers will find a dead animal that has been lying in the sun for days and eat it up—germs and all. They suffer no ill effects from this.

Dogs' and cats' digestive systems are not like that of humans. They are biologically designed to tolerate and even thrive on foods contaminated with bacteria. The stomach acids and enzymes in our pets are much stronger than ours, so they can eat things we couldn't touch, such as rotting dead flesh and animal feces—a primary source of E. coli and salmonella that sickens humans. Despite the fact that dogs put all sorts of unsanitary objects into their mouths and are exposed to large amounts of bacteria from these sources, they have far less bacteria living in their mouths than people do! This is because their saliva contains antibiotic substances that kill potentially harmful bacteria. Any bacteria that survive the saliva are killed by the powerful acids and enzymes in the dog's stomach.

The meats you bring home from the butcher are far cleaner than those they would find in the wild. If you are worried, you can always rinse the meat with water first. While this may not remove all possible contamination, it might make you feel better.

It is more dangerous feeding your pet dry kibble and the canned equivalents than fresh raw meats. Recalls occur all the time because of high levels of salmonella or some other biological or chemical contaminates in commercially prepared pet foods. Dogs eating kibble have a lower immune reaction to potential infection and, therefore, are much more prone to getting sick if they eat something that has a high level of some troublesome bacteria. Raw-fed dogs' immune systems are stronger and better able to fight off infection, which is another reason why raw-fed dogs and cats are less sickly overall.

MAKING THE CHANGE

Changing the diet can be confusing and hard at times for some pets. They get accustomed to eating a certain type of food and it may be a little difficult to get them to eat something totally different. This is true for raw foods as well.

If your pet has some experience eating a variety of home produced foods, both cooked and raw, a raw diet is more readily accepted and less likely to cause gastrointestinal disturbance than with an exclusively kibble-fed pet.

If you are making a transition from kibble or cheap canned foods to raw, start by feeding your dog or cat a higher quality, whole meat canned food. Make sure to add coconut oil so your pet benefits from eating the oil. Once your pet becomes used to having coconut oil in its food, the coconut oil provides a familiar taste when you transition to raw foods and he will be more likely to take to the change. After a couple of weeks on the canned food, add a little chopped raw meat. Mix it into the canned food along with the coconut oil. Gradually, increase the amount of raw foods while decreasing the canned food.

If your pet refuses to eat the canned food or the raw meat, consider a one or two day fast before feeding the food again. This will make your pet hungry enough to eat nearly anything and be more accepting of a change in its diet. Fasting will not harm your pet, it is a common occurrence in the wild and can be beneficial in allowing time for the digestive system to cleanse and detoxify. You can divide the daily meal into two smaller meals so that hunger is sustained and never completely satisfied at any one time. Otherwise, your pet may only eat part of the meal.

Dogs and cats love meat, particularly cooked meat. Animals prefer their meat to be cooked or aged over eating raw meat. In the wild they will immediately eat freshly killed prey because if they don't, they risk losing it to other animals. If they are not starving and do not have competition, they will reserve a kill and allow it to age a bit before eating it. Dogs will often burry a fresh kill and dig it up a week or so later to enjoy. Humans prefer aged meats as well. Butchers hang fresh beef for 2 to 3 weeks to allow it to age. This allows enzymes and lactic acids to break down the tissues, making the meat more tender and better tasting.

If you start feeding your pet meat that is partially cooked, he will take to it better than he would if it were completely raw. Over a period of several weeks you can cook the meat less and less until it is essentially raw. This way, your pet gradually gets used to eating raw meat.

THE EXPENSE

Some people may complain that feeding a pet with fresh meats and vegetables is too expensive. It may seem like that when you look at the grocery bill, but when you factor in all the savings from not going to the veterinarian and not buying a multitude of expensive medications and treatments, you will probably save money! Eating low quality pet foods, such as kibble, is the primary cause of the vast majority of health problems seen in our pets nowadays. Some people spend thousands of dollars to correct their pet's health problems, often without any significant improvement. A raw meat based diet can help to improve their health and their quality of life.

A natural or raw meat diet may not be as expensive as you might think. Foods for your cat or dog can be purchased economically. Ask the butcher for scraps, organs, necks, and backs. Often you can get them at a fraction of the price of regular cuts. Also, consider the meat sold at a discount because it has reached its best buy date. Simply because it is a few days older than the other meats doesn't make it unhealthy, and pets usually prefer the older meats! Buy vegetables when they are on sale. Most fresh vegetables are not that expensive anyway. You may also consider buying meats and vegetables in quantity when they are on sale and freezing the excess.

The biggest issue is time. You do need to spend a little extra time shopping for various ingredients, but usually you can get everything you need while you are shopping for yourself. What will take up most of your time is preparing the food. But you will have to decide if it is worth the time for your dog or cat to get nutritious food and be healthier.

If you just don't have the time to give, there are some sources of commercially prepared raw foods that are nutritionally balanced, as mentioned above. These products are available from pet and health food stores and many veterinarians. Of course, you will pay a little more for the convenience.

12

Healthy Foods and Recipes

GOING CUCKOO FOR COCONUT

Adding coconut products into your pet's diet can have a significant positive impact on its health, energy level, and appearance. Coconut oil, milk, meat, flour, and even water can be added to commercial and homemade meals to improve the nutritional content of your pet's food and to take advantage of the remarkable health properties of coconut oil. Because most pets love the taste of coconut, you can mix coconut oil into foods and medicines to make them more enticing to your pet. Please keep in mind that the recommendation of 1 teaspoon (5 ml) of coconut per 10 pounds (4.5 kg) of body weight is only a general guideline, not a strict rule. Coconut oil is a food, not a drug, so you can feed your pet more than this without harm. In fact, carnivorous animals like dogs and cats can tolerate a much higher amount of fat in their diet than humans can.

Coconut oil is extracted from coconut meat. Eating the meat itself will supply your pet with some of this beneficial oil. A 2 x 3-inch (5 x 8-cm) piece of fresh coconut meat contains about 1 tablespoon (15 ml) of coconut oil. Eating a 1 x 1-inch (2.5 x 2.5-cm) piece of fresh coconut would provide about 1 teaspoon.

Fresh coconuts are easy to find. They are sold in most grocery and health food stores. Opening a coconut can be a bit tricky. If you do it correctly, however, it can be done quickly and efficiently. In the islands, coconut sellers on street corners will hold the coconut in one hand and strike it sharply with the dull edge of a machete. With only one or two strikes the coconut splits in half. You can do the same without the danger of losing a finger. I suggest using a hammer and placing the coconut on the ground.

Before opening the coconut, you must first drain the water. Find the three "eyes" on the coconut and puncture two of them with an ice pick or hammer and nail. One of the eyes will be very soft and easy to puncture with the ice pick. The other two are a little harder

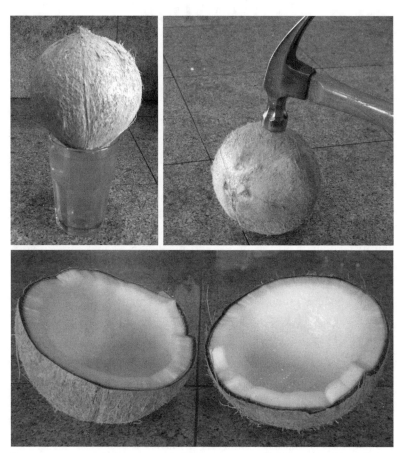

Puncture two of the eyes of the coconut and drain the liquid (top left). Strike the coconut on the equator (top right). The shell will split into two halves (bottom).

to puncture. Drain the coconut water completely. Once the water is out, put the coconut on a hard surface. The floor is better than the countertop because you will be hitting the coconut with a good deal of force. Hit the coconut on the equator, not on the eyes. When the coconut is hit on the equator, it will split in half fairly easily with just a couple of blows. At this stage, the shell is easier to break into smaller pieces. Large pieces of coconut shell, with the meat still attached, can be given to your dog and he will chew on it like a bone. Coconut meat can be pried off the shell with a knife. You will notice a thin layer of brown skin on the side of the meat that was attached to the shell. You can leave this on, it is totally edible. You can store unused coconut in an air tight container in the refrigerator for about five days or in the freezer for several months.

Your dog will love fresh coconut, but buying a package of dried, unsweetened desiccated coconut is a lot less trouble. When fresh coconut is shredded and dried, only the water is removed; all the oil remains. Dried shredded or flaked coconut can provide just as much coconut oil as fresh coconut. Actually, since the water is removed, the same weight of dried coconut will contain more coconut oil than fresh coconut. One cup of fresh shredded coconut contains 27 grams (about 2 tablespoons) of coconut oil. A cup of dried shredded coconut contains 50 grams (about 3½ tablespoons) of coconut oil.

Coconut milk provides another source of coconut oil. Coconut milk is made by shredding then crushing the juice out of coconut meat. This juice is coconut milk. Coconut oil manufacturers often extract the oil from fresh coconut milk. It is fairly easy to do. The simplest method is to put the milk in a container and let it sit for about 36 hours. Oil, being lighter than water, will float to the surface and collect on top. If you put the container into the refrigerator, this layer of oil will harden, which will allow you to pick it up and remove it from the watery portion.

When manufacturers make coconut milk, they leave the oil in the milk. You can buy coconut milk in most grocery and health food stores. It is usually sold in 14 ounce (400 ml) cans. One can of coconut milk contains about 5 tablespoons of coconut oil. Cats and dogs love the taste of coconut milk. The best tasting and healthiest coconut milk, without fillers, sugars, or preservatives, is homemade.

HOW TO MAKE YOUR OWN COCONUT MILK

You can make coconut milk in one of two ways—from fresh coconuts or from dried shredded coconut. Both ways are described below.

Coconut Milk from Fresh Coconut

Pierce two eyes of a coconut and drain the liquid. Crack open the coconut and remove the white meat. Pry the meat off the shell. The meat will have a thin brown layer where it was attached to the shell. You do not need to remove this layer. Cut the meat into about 1-inch (2.5 cm) pieces. Place the meat into a blender along with just enough hot water to cover the coconut. The less water you use, the creamier the resulting milk will be. Blend until the coconut is finely chopped.

Place several layers of cheesecloth in a strainer. Pour the coconut mixture through the cheesecloth and strainer, collecting the liquid in a bowl. Wrap the cheesecloth around the shredded coconut, and with your hands squeeze as much of the liquid out of the meat as possible. This is your first squeezing or pressing. The resulting liquid is very rich and creamy. If you like, you can put the coconut back into the blender with a little more hot water and repeat the process to extract a little more milk. The second pressing will yield a slightly less rich milk.

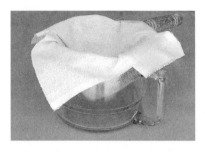
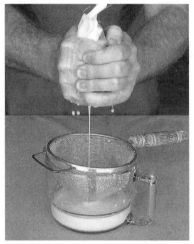

Pour the coconut mixture into the cheese cloth (left). Squeeze out the remaining liquid (right).

156

Discard the shredded coconut or use it as you would shredded coconut. This shredded coconut also makes good birdfeed. Use the milk immediately or store in the refrigerator. The milk should be used within about three days.

Coconut Milk from Dried Coconut

Empty an 8 ounce package of unsweetened, unsulfured shredded coconut into a blender. Add 1 cup of hot water. Blend for about 30 seconds and allow the mixture a few minutes to cool.

Place several layers of cheesecloth in a strainer. Pour the coconut mixture through the cheesecloth and strainer, collecting the liquid in a bowl. Wrap the cheesecloth around the shredded coconut and with your hands squeeze as much of the liquid out of the meat as possible. This is your first squeezing or pressing. You can put the coconut back into the blender with a little more hot water and repeat the process to extract a little more milk.

Discard the coconut and store the coconut milk in the refrigerator. Use within three days.

BUILDING STRONG BONES AND TEETH
Fresh Bones

We hear a lot about the importance of calcium in building strong bones and preventing osteoporosis, but there is much more to bones than just calcium. While calcium is the major mineral in bones, it is not the only mineral. Taking calcium supplements alone will not build better bones. Magnesium, boron, silicon, manganese, and other minerals as well as vitamin D and fat are also essential in the bone building process. Without all of these other minerals and nutrients, calcium is useless in bone building. In fact, feeding your pet calcium supplements without magnesium and other minerals can actually weaken the bones.

The best source of all the minerals needed for bone building is found in bones themselves. Feeding your pet bones in some form will provide the exact materials needed in the exact proportions needed. Eating and chewing on bones provides the perfect combination and ratio of minerals for bone building. Exposure to an adequate amount of sunlight provides the vitamin D and coconut oil can provide the

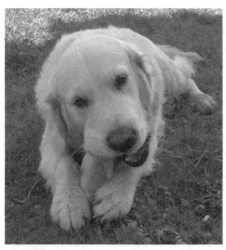

Golden Retriever chewing on a bone.

needed fat. Fat is necessary because it improves the absorption of calcium and other minerals. Coconut oil has shown to do these better than other fats.

In addition to providing a source of minerals, chewing on large raw meaty bones helps strengthen the jaw muscles, cleans the teeth, and provides a source of enjoyment and a tasty activity. Leaving a little meat on the bone enhances the enjoyment. Raw bones are preferred because cooking causes bones to become brittle and splinter, which can lead to choking or injury. This is the reason for the well known warning not to feed your dog cooked chicken bones. Even though chicken bones are small, when they are cooked they become stiff and brittle. Cats and even dogs eat bones in rodents and birds all the time without problem because these raw bones are softer and more chewable.

Dogs readily take to chewing on fresh bones, cats not so much. Yet cats still need their minerals. Whole raw bones are not the only good source of minerals. Below are a few other options that work just as well and perhaps even better.

Bone Meal

Bone meal is made from defatted, dried, and flash-frozen animal bones that are ground to a powder. Adding bone meal to dog and cat food is another way to incorporate minerals into your pet's diet.

However, you need to be careful where you purchase bone meal. Buy it from a pet store and read the label to ensure it is meant specifically for animal consumption. Do not use the bone meal sold at home and garden stores, as this product is developed for fertilizing plants and is toxic to your dog or cat.

The simplest way to give it to your pet is to just mix a half spoonful or so in its food. You can make a treat for your pet by mixing a little bone meal with coconut oil and putting it into the refrigerator to harden. Cut the hardened coconut oil into serving sizes suitable for your pet and feed it to him as a treat. Adding coconut oil or other fat to the bone meal is important in order for it to be properly absorbed. Otherwise it is just going to go in and out without much benefit.

Eggshell Powder

Eggshells are another excellent source of bone building minerals. In addition to calcium, they contain magnesium, boron, copper, iron, manganese, molybdenum, sulfur, silicon, zinc and at least 17 others. The composition of eggshell is very similar to that of bone and provides an excellent source of minerals for building strong, healthy bones and teeth. Studies have shown that ground eggshells added to animal's diets can significantly improve bone mineral density.

Save your eggshells, rinse them out and let them dry. You can keep them in the refrigerator for several days and accumulate them. Break them into fingernail size pieces and spread them out on an oven safe dish or cookie sheet. Preheat the oven to 300 degrees F (150 C or gas mark 2). Bake the shells for about 30 minutes. This process kills bacteria and completely dries them out so that they are easier to pulverize. Remove them from the oven and let cool.

Put a handful (about ¼ cup) of the eggshells in a coffee grinder. Any coffee grinder will do, even inexpensive ones do a good job. Grind the shells until they are completely powdered, about 10 seconds. Remove them from the grinder and store in a bottle or other sealed container. Store it in the cupboard and use as needed.

Like bone meal, eggshell powder can be mixed into your pet's food or made into a treat using coconut oil. See description above.

Bone Broth

Bone broth is a mineral rich soup stock made by boiling bones in water with a little vinegar. The vinegar acidifies the water slightly, allowing more minerals to be leached from the bones. Sometimes vegetables are added, but are optional. Bone broth supplies all the minerals needed to build strong bones and teeth. Both humans and pets can benefit from eating it. The broth can be consumed as a savory beverage, your dog or cat will love it, or it can be used in preparing other foods, such as the hearty meat and vegetable stew described later in this chapter.

In addition to strengthening bones and teeth, bone broth is also good for connective tissues, cartilage, ligaments, joints, hair, skin, and claws due to its high collagen content. It provides nutrients necessary to build and maintain healthy joint function and prevent arthritis.

You can use any type of bone and cartilage to make the broth—beef, lamb, pork, chicken, fish, and others. Include the cartilage around the ends of the bones. Save leftover bones from family meals. Use all your leftover chicken bones, gristle, and skin; don't throw them away. You can get ox tail, soup bones, knuckles, and other bones from your butcher or local grocer. Often times you can get them for free or for a minimal charge. I buy chicken backs from our health foods store's butcher shop for almost nothing. These chicken backs are loaded with bones, cartilage, skin, and even meat. Large beef, pork, and lamb bones with cartilage attached are some of the best to use. Cartilage is easier to dissolve than hard bone and quickly enriches the broth. Larger bones are filled with nutrient-rich bone marrow. Make sure long bones are cut in half and scrape all the marrow out of them before removing them from the cooked broth. Marrow has a soft, fatty-like consistency. Mash it up and stir it into the broth.

Bone broth is easy and inexpensive to make. Begin by putting the bones into a pot and filling the pot with water. Use just enough water to cover the bones by about 1 inch (2.5 cm). For each pint or 2 cups (240 ml) of water used, add 1 to 2 teaspoons of apple cider vinegar. Vegetables such as carrots, celery, and herbs can be added but are optional. Do not use onions or garlic, as they can cause problems for your pet (see Foods You Should Never Feed Your Pet at the end of the chapter). Bring the water to a rolling boil, reduce the heat, and let it simmer for about 8 to 12 hours. Keep the broth covered while cooking. If necessary, you may add a little water to keep the bones submerged. I suggest adding a little unrefined sea salt to enhance the flavor and add the benefit of trace minerals from the salt. Cool the broth before using. You can make plenty at one time and store it in the refrigerator for up to 6 days or freeze it for up to 6 months or more.

If your broth included a lot of cartilage, it may become somewhat thick or gelatinous when chilled. You can thin it down with a little water. Heating it slightly will also liquefy it. Bone broth can be given to your pet like you would a cup of water. They will lap it up in no time. It goes well mixed into other foods to increase flavor and moisture content. It also makes a good base for the hearty meat and vegetable stew described below.

HEARTY MEAT AND VEGETABLE STEW (STOMACH STEW)

I call this "stomach stew" because it mimics the nutrients carnivores get in the wild when they eat the internal organs and stomach contents of their prey.

The best diet for your pet is a natural one—one that they would eat in the wild if given the opportunity. Dogs are scavengers, although they will eat any small animal they can catch. Cats and ferrets are obligate carnivores—they must have a meat-based diet. Cats are natural born hunters. You see them at play stalking insects or small rodents, acting just like their big cousins in Africa stalking gazelles and wildebeests. After a kill, lions, tigers, hyenas, wolves, and other carnivorous animals in the wild will eat the insides of the prey first. The muscle meat and bones come last. They relish organ meats and especially the stomach and its contents, which are the most nutritious parts of the animal.

The stomachs of herbivores and omnivores contain essentially the only source of vegetable matter in carnivores' diets. Lions and wolves and their domestic counterparts—cats and dogs—do not have the proper digestive system to completely digest vegetable matter. Their digestive tract is designed for raw meat. It is much shorter than that of herbivores, so food is transported quickly. In herbivores, vegetable matter is passed slowly through a long gastrointestinal tract to ensure nutrients are adequately extracted. Some animals (cows, deer, antelope, sheep, etc.) have multiple stomachs so that hard to digest vegetable matter can be broken down to yield as much nutrition as possible. Partially digested food called the cud is regurgitated and chewed again to break down the fiber (cellulose) even further. Many herbivores secrete special cellulose digesting enzymes that can break down the tough cell walls. Cats and dogs don't have this type of digestive system and don't have cellulose digestive enzymes and so cannot digest vegetable matter very well. Cows will chew their food, regurgitate it, and chew it again, extracting as much of the nutrition as possible. The carnivore jaw does not allow for the sideways movement that the herbivore jaws possess, but only an up and down action, perfect for ripping and tearing apart meat and bone. Cats and dogs don't chew their food; they rip it into bite size pieces and swallow it whole. Protein and fat digesting enzymes do the majority of the job of breaking the meat down to release its nutrients. Most raw vegetable matter goes in and out of carnivores without being completely broken down, providing little nutrition.

Herbivores and omnivores can benefit from eating raw plant foods; carnivores cannot. Plant eating animals have the digestive system and enzymes to handle raw plant foods. The only plant foods carnivores can benefit from are those that are already partially digested in the digestive tracts of their prey. This plant material has already been masticated and broken down by digestive enzymes before it is eaten by the carnivore.

When meat, milk, and eggs, are cooked, the proteins in them are denatured and become harder to digest, and therefore less nutritious. Heat alters protein structure. You can visibly see this every time you fry an egg. During cooking, the egg white transforms from a clear liquid (which is very easy to digest) to a white rubbery texture, which is harder to digest. The longer the meat is cooked, the harder it is to digest and the more vitamins are lost. This is why dogs, cats, and other carnivorous pets do better with a raw meat diet.

Dogs and cats love to drink milk. However, pasteurized milk is not the best source of nourishment. Pasteurization is done to kill any potentially harmful bacteria that may contaminate the milk. In the process, good bacteria that promote healthy digestive function are also killed. It's the good bacteria that allow the milk to ferment and even protect it from the effects of harmful bacteria. Pasteurized milk, as it gets old, does not ferment—it putrefies and spoils. In the past, if you wanted soured (raw) milk that you could drink and enjoy, all you had to do was leave it out on the countertop. Nowadays if you did that, you would get rotten milk with a horrible stench. The difference between the two is that raw milk is a living food with good bacteria; pasteurized milk is dead and slowly rotting, and if not refrigerated, the rate at which it rots accelerates.

Infants thrive on their mothers' milk as their sole source of nourishment for the first months of life. Milk is often referred to as the perfect food because it supplies all the nutrients an infant needs during this period. The same is true for every mammal. When milk is pasteurized, some of nutrients are lost, good bacteria are killed, proteins are denatured, and fats are oxidized, making the product far less nutritious. Although the basic nutrient content is similar between raw and pasteurized milk, the quality of the milk and of the nutrients is very different. Studies have shown that feeding newborn calves pasteurized cow's milk in place of raw milk has a pronounced detrimental effect on growth and development. Dr. Pottenger's studies showed the same thing. Cats raised on pasteurized milk failed to thrive, while those that ate raw cow's milk developed normally and healthfully. Carnivorous animals, like dogs and cats, need raw animal-derived foods (meat, milk, eggs) for optimal health.

However, when vegetables or plant foods are cooked they become softer and easier to digest and generally more nutritious. Let me explain why. All the vitamins and minerals are found in the fluids inside the plant's cells. Each cell is encapsulated by a tough cell wall that is made of a sturdy fibrous material called cellulose. In order to access the nutrients, the cell wall must be broken open. This is normally accomplished by chewing or by the action of cellulose digesting enzymes in the gut. Another way to break open the cell wall is by heating. When plants are cooked to the point of boiling, the nutrient rich fluid inside the cells expands, causing the cell to burst open, releasing the nutrients. This is why the water used for boiling vegetables can be more nutritious than the vegetables themselves.

Doesn't cooking destroy the nutrients? There is some loss but the benefits of low to moderate cooking override the tiny loss of some of the vitamins. Minerals are not affected by heat, so there is no loss there. Most vitamins are also not affected much by heat. The percentage of heat sensitive vitamins that are lost depends on the cooking temperature and the length of time. Exposure to high heat for extended periods of time can destroy about 50 percent of vitamins B_1, A, C, and E. But short duration, low temperature cooking will have a minimal effect. Vegetables only need to be heated to boiling and simmered for about 5-10 minutes. Hard root vegetables need to be cooked a little longer than softer vegetables. Leafy greens need only a minute or two. Because cooking releases nutrients from the plant cells, overall nutritional value actually increases.

Stomach stew is a meat and vegetable stew made with bone broth, vegetables, fat, and meat. The purpose of the stew is to mimic the nutritional composition of the stomach contents (partially digested vegetables) and internal organs (organ meats and fat) that carnivores get from hunting and eating wild prey. The stomachs of herbivores are usually filled with partially digested grass and leaves. Stomach stew is made using higher quality vegetables that provide a much greater amount of vitamins and minerals. When a variety of different vegetables and meats (including organ meats) are used, stomach stew provides a complete and balanced diet for your pet.

The vegetables in the stew are chopped and boiled until slightly soft to simulate the partially digested vegetable matter in a prey animal's stomach. You may put the vegetables in a blender to chop them finer if desired, but they still need to be cooked because the blender will not chop them fine enough to break all the cell walls. Fat trimmed from meat is added while cooking to flavor the stew. Coconut oil and meat are added at the end and the stew is removed from the heat and allowed to cool. The meat should be cut into bite size pieces and constitute at least half of the bulk of the stew. Eggs and raw or fermented dairy may also be added. When all the ingredients are combined, the stew should be thick and chunky, not watery.

Enough of the vegetable broth can be made at one time to last for two or three days. Each day a serving portion can we warmed and combined with fresh meat and other animal products before serving. The combination of ingredients should vary. Use different types of vegetables and meats. Emphasize organ meats over muscle meats. Add raw eggs and raw or fermented dairy occasionally. A source of fat must always be included, preferably coconut oil, meat fat, red palm oil, or raw cream. A little olive oil is fine occasionally.

Avoid using grains and high-carb vegetables such as potatoes (see list below). People often like to give their pets fruits because to us, they taste good. But dogs and cats have different tastes. Cats can't even taste sweetness, so fruit isn't all that appealing to them. Fruit is often high in sugar and other carbohydrates and is not recommended. Limit the use of medium-carb vegetables. Since excessive carbohydrate consumption can lead to many health problems, it is best to keep carbohydrate consumption low. Carnivores thrive on protein and fat and have little need for carbohydrate and absolutely no need for sugar or sweets. Keeping in mind these guidelines, below is a list of possible foods that could be used in making stomach stew. This list does not include all possible foods you can use, but serves as a general guide.

Carbohydrate (Vegetable) Sources

High-Carb Vegetables:
White potatoes
Beans (pinto, black, red, etc.)
Grains (wheat, rice, barley, etc,)
Soy
Fruits

Medium-Carb Vegetables:
Winter squash (acorn, butternut,
  pumpkin, etc.)
Sweet potato
Yam
Carrot
Beet
Turnip
Parsnip

Low-Carb Vegetables:
Summer squash
Broccoli
Brussels sprouts
Cabbage
Cauliflower
Celery
Green beans
Peas
Coconut meat (fresh or dried)
Asparagus
Spinach
Kale

Kelp
Fennel
Bell pepper
Tomato
Eggplant
Chard
Bok choy
Napa cabbage
Lettuce
Beet greens
Collard greens
Sauerkraut

Protein Sources	Fat Sources
Beef	Coconut oil
Fowl (chicken, turkey, etc.)	Coconut milk
Pork	Red palm oil
Lamb	Extra virgin olive oil
Goat	Meat fat/drippings
Fish	Butter
Game meats (deer, elk, etc.)	Raw cream
Gelatin	
Eggs	
Organ meats (tongue, heart, liver, kidneys, tripe, etc.)	
Raw whole milk (cow, goat)	
Fermented, unsweetened whole milk (yogurt or kefir)	
Cheese	

All meats, eggs, and milk should be raw. In many of the states in the US, it is illegal to sell raw milk for human consumption, so raw milk may be hard to find in these locations even when it is legal for pets to consume. You can find sources for raw milk at this website: www.realmilk.com. You don't need to worry about raw milk being contaminated by harmful bacteria. Dairy farms that process raw milk follow strict sanitary standards and their milk is safer to drink than pasteurized milk. People and animals have consumed raw milk for generations without worrying about bacteria. Contaminated pasteurized milk, however, is a much greater concern because pasteurized milk doesn't have the good bacteria to prevent the bad bacteria from growing. Raw milk is actually considered a health food because of all the good bacteria it contains, so giving your pet unpasteurized raw milk or fermented milk from a reliable source should not be a concern.

In the stew, use both the typical muscle meats you find at the grocer as well as a variety of organ meats. Some will be sold along with other fresh cuts of meat. You may also ask the butcher for others.

Gelatin is made from collagen obtained from various animal by-products. It is what Jell-O is made from. You can buy powdered gelatin without sugar or flavoring. Gelatin is a rich source of protein and can be added to the stew to increase the protein content.

Raw eggs provide a very nutritious source of protein, vitamins, minerals, and fats. They also add flavor that dogs and cats enjoy, making the stomach stew more enticing. Eggs are a powerhouse of nutrition. They supply a high-quality protein with a full range of essential amino acids. Eggs also contain a wide spectrum of important nutrients such as vitamins A, D, B_6, B_{12}, thiamin, riboflavin, niacin, and choline; minerals calcium, magnesium, potassium, zinc, and selenium; and essential fatty acids, including the omega-3 fatty acid DHA.

Some people have expressed concerns about giving raw eggs to pets. One concern is the fear of salmonella poisoning. If you use organic or free-range eggs and wash the shell first, there is no threat of salmonella. Salmonella contamination has only been reported in eggs from factory farms where chickens are confined to small cages, stacked on top of each other, living under filthy, unhealthy conditions. Free-range chickens are allowed to go out into the sunlight and graze, eating and living more like they would in the wild. Consequently, they are much healthier and so are their eggs.

Another concern is the presence of avidin, a protein in raw egg white. Avidin binds to biotin, one of the B vitamins, preventing it from being completely absorbed into the body. Consumption of raw eggs over a long period of time can increase the risk of a biotin deficiency. Fortunately, the needs for biotin are low and many foods provide adequate amounts of it. It is also synthesized by bacteria in the intestinal tract. Adding 3 or 4 raw eggs a week to the stomach stew is not likely to cause any problems. However, if you are concerned, you can separate the egg whites from the yolks and add the whites to the stew during the last few minutes as it is cooking. Exposure to just 4 minutes in simmering hot water will completely deactivate avidin's biotin binding capability. After removing the stew from the stove and allowing it to cool, you can add the raw egg yolk.

Fermented foods such as sauerkraut, yogurt, and kefir make healthy additions to the stomach stew. They should always be added after cooking, when the stew is at or near room temperature. These foods should contain live bacteria cultures and should be without added sugar or flavorings. Fermentation breaks down proteins making them easier to digest and restores many of the enzymes destroyed during cooking. Fermentation also improves nutrient content, especially boosting the B vitamins. The fermenting bacteria also help support and repopulate the good bacteria in the digestive tract that are important to good digestive function.

Do not skimp on the fat. Fats are essential for your pet's health. Stomach stew should be rich in fat.

Basic Stew Recipe

The stew should be made fresh each day. However, to conserve your time you can keep a portion of the vegetable broth and store it in the refrigerator for the following day or two. Just heat and add meat, fat, and any other ingredients desired.

The choice of vegetables, protein, and fat used is up to you. You can make any combination you desire. This also allows you to be creative and add variety to your pet's meals. Generally it is best to keep it simple and not try to use too many ingredients for any one stew.

No measurements are specified here because that will change depending on how much you make. If you have a Chihuahua you will make a smaller amount than if you had a Saint Bernard. Likewise, if you have two or three dogs or cats you will make more than if you just had one. You don't need exact measurements; just make the amount that your pet will eat without overfeeding it.

This recipe includes 1 hard, 1 medium, and 1 soft vegetable (carrot, zucchini, spinach), but it could include any combination of vegetables or just a single vegetable. The meat could be any cut of muscle or organ meat. The skin of chicken and other fowl should also be added when these meats are used. The skin can add flavor to the stew and should be added at the beginning and cooked with the vegetables. The following is an example of how to make the stew.

Ingredients:
Water or bone broth
Beef fat
Carrot, cut into bite size pieces
Zucchini, sliced
Spinach, chopped
Raw beef, cut into bite size pieces
Coconut oil
Dash sea salt
Raw or fermented dairy (optional)

Put water or bone broth in a 1 quart (1 liter) saucepan. If you use water to make the stew instead of bone broth, add some bone meal or eggshell powder to the stew. You don't need much, ¼ teaspoon per serving will do. For example, if you have a medium size dog (20-60 pounds/10-30 kg), and are making only one serving (one meal), use ¼ teaspoon. Adjust the amount for larger or smaller dogs and cats and for multiple servings.

Add beef fat and carrot (hard vegetable) and bring to a boil, reduce heat and simmer for about 10 minutes. Add zucchini (medium vegetable) and simmer for another 5-10 minutes. Add spinach (leafy green or soft vegetable) and simmer 1 to 2 minutes. Add meat, coconut oil, and salt. Turn off the heat and remove the pan from the stove. The meat should comprise at least half the bulk of the stew. You can rinse off the raw meat with a little water under the facet if you like before adding it to the stew. Adding raw meat to the hot stew will kill any bacteria on the surface of the meat, where it is most likely to be, and make it tastier to your dog or cat, but still leave the inside completely raw. Let the stew cool to about room temperature or just slightly warm.

After the stew has cooled, you can add eggs, raw milk, yogurt, or other dairy if you like. Sauerkraut and other fermented vegetables could be added at this time as well. You don't want to cook sauerkraut or yogurt as it will kill the beneficial bacteria they contain. Adding one or two of these foods greatly increases the nutritional content of the stew and its palatability.

Transition Stew

If your pet is not accustomed to eating raw meat or organ meats, it may not take to the stew immediately. In this case, transition stew is useful. This stew helps transition your pet from commercial foods to raw meat stomach stew. Transition stew is made with the same ingredients, but the meat is cooked slightly. Cooking the meat makes the stew more palatable and enticing to dogs and cats. Follow the directions above for making the stew, but after adding the meat continue to simmer the stew for several minutes to cook the meat. This will release meat juices into the stew and make it more flavorful. Before serving, adding raw milk, yogurt, kefir, cheese, coconut milk, or eggs to the stew will also make it more enticing.

Unless your dog or cat is already used to eating raw organ meat, I recommend everyone start out with the transition stew. Once your dog or cat gets used to eating this version of the stomach stew, you can gradually reduce the cooking time of the meat.

If your dog or cat is currently eating kibble, you will need to transition him to canned food first. After several weeks of canned food, try the transition stew. If your cat or dog is still hesitant about eating the stew or only eats part of it, mix in a little of the canned food he is used to eating. Adding eggs and milk will also help. If he is still picky, let him fast for a day or two with just water but without any food. He will start eating the stew.

FOODS YOU SHOULD NEVER FEED YOUR PET

There are certain foods you should never feed your pet or use in homemade pet food. Foods that lack good nutrition and are not particularly healthy for people are not any healthier for our pets. There is no place in your pet's diet for junk foods such as potato chips, cookies, donuts, soda, pizza, frozen dinners, and other convenience and snack foods. While eating these types of foods on rare occasions is not particularly harmful, there are foods that we eat all the time that can cause real damage and can even be fatal to your pet. These foods should never be given to your dog or cat or any pet for that matter. Some of these foods, like candy and gum, are obviously not good dietary choices for humans or pets; others such as avocados and grapes that are generally considered healthy for us are not good for our pets.

Chocolate

Chocolate contains a toxic substance called theobromine. Humans can metabolize theobromine without too much problem, but many animals cannot. The most common victims of theobromine poisoning are dogs who will readily eat chocolate if given the chance. Symptoms many include vomiting, abnormal heart rhythm, tremors, seizures, and death. Cats are even more sensitive to theobromine poisoning, but they are less likely to eat chocolate because they are unable to taste sweetness. Although cats usually won't eat chocolate if given the choice, they can be coaxed into it by owners who think they are giving the cat a treat. All forms of chocolate are dangerous, including white chocolate. Dark chocolate and unsweetened baker's chocolate contain more theobromine than milk chocolate. Raw cacao beans, a popular natural treat from which chocolate is made, contain the most.

Candy and Gum

Candy is a source of empty calories that supplies no nutritional benefit whatsoever. In addition, it can adversely affect blood sugar and promote weight gain, diabetes, heart problems, and dementia. Sugar-free candy may not contain sugar but can be just as bad, if not worse. Xylitol, a non-caloric sweetener used in sugar-free candy, gum, toothpaste, and baked goods, can cause more trouble than sugar. In dogs and cats it can increase insulin levels, which will cause blood sugar to drop, leading to hypoglycemia. Acute symptoms may include vomiting, lethargy, loss of coordination and possibly seizures. Reportedly, consuming xylitol over a period of just a few days can lead to liver failure.

Avocado

Avocados and guacamole can be a healthy choice for us, but for our pets they can turn deadly. Avocados contain a fungicidal toxin called persin. Persin leaches into the fruit from the pit and the skin, making the entire fruit inedible for many animals. Humans are generally immune to its effects, but dogs, cats, and other domestic animals are not. Symptoms of persin poisoning may include vomiting, diarrhea, abnormal heart rate, labored breathing, and even death.

Macadamia Nuts

Macadamia nuts are often found in cookies, candies, and other treats. While they may taste delicious, they are not good for our pets. Dogs, for example, may suffer from a series of symptoms after consumption of macadamia nuts, which include weakness or paralysis of the hindquarters, rapid heart rate, elevated body temperature, and vomiting. As few as six raw or roasted macadamia nuts can make a dog ill. Eating chocolate covered macadamia nuts will make symptoms worse, possibly leading to death.

Grapes and Raisins

Veterinarians aren't sure why, but these fruits can induce kidney failure in dogs and cats. Even eating just a couple may cause problems, especially in small dogs and cats. Although some pets appear to show no ill effects, you can't always tell what degree of damage the fruit may be causing, especially if they are given in small quantities over a long period of time. It would be wise not to keep grapes and raisins on countertops or other places that may be accessible to your pets in case they try to eat them without your knowledge.

Onions and Garlic

Plants in the onion (Allium) family, which includes onions, garlic, chives, scallions, leeks, and shallots, are often used to season our foods and are known to have health benefits to humans, but they can wreck havoc on our pets. Members of the onion family contain sulfoxides that are harmless to us but toxic to cats, dogs, guinea pigs, chickens, parrots, and many other animals. Sulfoxides can cause gastrointestinal irritation and damage red blood cells, leading to anemia.

Onions and garlic in all forms—raw, cooked, dehydrated, and powdered—are dangerous. Because onions and garlic are commonly added to commercially prepared foods, it is wise not to feed your pets human foods from the grocery store or leftovers brought home from a restaurant such as leftover pizza, Chinese food, canned spaghetti, frozen dinners, and such. Even prepared baby food may contain onion powder.

Dried Fruit

When fruit is dried, most of the water is removed, leaving a smaller volume of food with a higher concentration of sugar. Feeding your pet raisins, dates, prunes, and other dried fruits is the same as feeding them candy. In fact, it can be worse than candy. The sticky dried fruit tends to cling onto and between teeth where it sits and rots. Sugars in the fruit cause bacteria overgrowth, which can lead to tooth decay, gum disease, and bad breath.

Birds can handle dried fruit better than most other pets. Because they have beaks, there are no teeth for the fruit to stick on to and